The Biopolitics of Beauty

The Biopolitics of Beauty

Cosmetic Citizenship and Affective Capital in Brazil

Alvaro Jarrín

UNIVERSITY OF CALIFORNIA PRESS

University of California Press, one of the most
distinguished university presses in the United States,
enriches lives around the world by advancing scholarship
in the humanities, social sciences, and natural sciences. Its
activities are supported by the UC Press Foundation and
by philanthropic contributions from individuals and
institutions. For more information, visit www.ucpress.edu.

University of California Press
Oakland, California

Chapter 2 is based on the following article: Alvaro E.
Jarrin, "The Rise of the Cosmetic Nation: Plastic
Governmentality and Hybrid Medical Practices in Brazil,"
Medical Anthropology 31, no. 3 (2012): 213–228,
reproduced with permission from Taylor & Francis.

Chapter 4 is based on the following essay: Alvaro E.
Jarrin, "Favela Models: Sexual Virtue and Hopeful
Narratives of Beauty in Brazil," in Girls' Sexualities and
the Media, edited by Kate Harper, Yasmina Katsulis,
Vera Lopez, and Georganne Scheiner Gillis (New York:
Peter Lang, 2013), ISBN: 9781433122767, reproduced
with permission from the editors and Peter Lang.

Library of Congress Cataloging-in-Publication Data

Names: Jarrín, Alvaro, 1980- author.
Title: The biopolitics of beauty : cosmetic citizenship and
    affective capital in Brazil / Alvaro Jarrín.
Description: Oakland, California : University of
    California Press, [2017] | Includes bibliographical
    references and index.
Identifiers: LCCN 2017006866| ISBN 9780520293878
    (cloth : alk. paper) | ISBN 9780520293885 (pbk. : alk.
    paper) | ISBN 9780520967212 (ebook)
Subjects: LCSH: Surgery, Plastic—Social aspects—Brazil. |
    Biopolitics—Brazil. | Public health--Social aspects—
    Brazil. | Plastic surgeons—Social aspects—Brazil. |
    Beauty, Personal—Social aspects--Brazil.
Classification: LCC RD119 .J37 2017 | DDC 617.9/
    50981—dc23
LC record available at https://lccn.loc.gov/2017006866

Contents

Illustrations

Acknowledgments

It is impossible to put into words how many people have helped me along the winding road of writing this book. In many ways, this book is not solely mine but has depended on the labor and care of others, who made the research possible in the first place and who were there for me during the long research and writing process.

I thank all the people in Brazil who were willing to befriend me, spend some time talking to a young anthropologist, and provide me with a glimpse into their lives, hopes, and struggles. This book would have been impossible without their patient collaboration, and I hope I have done justice to their stories and their commitment to beauty. I am also thankful for the academic interlocutors who were willing to provide me with a host institution at which to present my work, especially the scholars who were part of the Programa Avançado de Cultura Contemporânea at UFRJ, and those who participated in the Laboratório de Etnografia e Estudos de Comunicação, Cultura e Cognição at UFF.

My fieldwork buddies, Beatriz Rodriguez Balanta, Lucia Cantero, and Bryan Pitts, have not only been partners in crime in Rio de Janeiro and São Paulo but have also helped me think through many of the issues this book addresses. The panels we put together, the papers we cowrote, and the feedback we gave on each other's work have been central to my understanding of Brazil's ongoing inequalities and political upheavals.

I am grateful for the generous intellectual community at Duke University that cultivated this project in its initial stages, and for the lasting friendships that have provided continuous support and feedback during more than a decade of research and writing. Anne Allison, Diane Nelson, and Rebecca Stein have been incredibly dedicated mentors throughout the whole process, especially during the grueling job search that eventually provided me with the financial stability to write. Margot Weiss and Leigh Campoamor have been selfless with their time, providing invaluable feedback for two chapters in the book, and Bianca Williams helped me write the book proposal that led to this book.

I rewrote the conclusion to this book after attending the "Politics of Beauty" conference at the University of Cambridge, and I am very thankful to the organizers and all the participants, particularly Marcia Ochoa, Mimi Thi Nguyen, Sarah Banet-Weiser, Shirley Tate, Rosemarie Garland-Thomson, and Mónica Moreno-Figueroa, for helping me refine my critique of Judith Butler and rethink the transnational implications of my work. Among other readers of this work are good friends like Jason Roberge, Paul Christensen, Ellis Jones, Nadine Knight, and several members of the Latin American and Latino Studies program at the College of the Holy Cross, including Melissa Weiner, Maria Rodrigues, Rosa Carrasquillo, Antonia Carcelén and Jorge Santos, among many others.

I am so thankful for reviewers of my work whom I have never met in person, but who nonetheless provided detailed feedback on how to improve the manuscript for this book. Robin Sheriff, Erica Lorraine Williams, and one other, anonymous reviewer were particularly generous with their fantastic suggestions, and I thank them for their dedication. My editor, Reed Malcolm, gave me invaluable pointers as I prepared the manuscript, and everyone else at the University of California Press made the process of putting this manuscript into print incredibly straightforward. I am especially thankfully to Bonita Hurd for her excellent copyediting work and to Cynthia Savage for crafting the index.

I thank Vincent Rosenblatt for providing fantastic photographs for the manuscript, as well as all the other people who provided permission to reproduce their work.

This book would not have been possible without the financial support of several academic programs and granting agencies. I was able to carry out my research and writing as a result of the generous support of the Wenner-Gren Foundation; the UNC/Duke Consortium for Latin American and Caribbean Studies; the Gender, Sexuality and Feminist Studies program at Duke; the Mellon/ACLS Early Career Fellowship Program; and a Batchelor-Ford Summer Fellowship at Holy Cross.

My friends and family were always there for me, and they rooted for my success through thick and thin. My dear Williams Goodrich Gang—you all have a special place in my heart, and I am so glad for your friendship. My awesome siblings—thanks for always supporting my studies and believing in my potential from a very young age. Mamita—you taught me to persevere no matter the circumstances, and to be true to myself. I admire your strength so much, and I am so very lucky that I inherited it.

This book is dedicated to my father, who taught me the love of books when I was very young. I remember fondly how much he enjoyed buying books for me and sharing our glimpses into other ways of life in the pages of a novel or a nonfiction book. It was through books that I became a critical thinker and became fascinated with human behavior, and it was that fascination that eventually led me to discover anthropology—the discipline that seeks to gather the stories of others and make sense of why people do the things they do. I wish my father were alive to see that I, too, can generate insights into human beings and their puzzling behavior.

Last, but certainly not least, I thank my husband and the love of my life, Fox Jarrín, for making sure I stopped working in the evenings, for feeding me delicious meals, for combating my constant self-doubt, and for generally taking care of me throughout the whole writing process. Fox, I feel this book owes much to you and your ability to make me happy, and I am so glad that we have made a home together. I am sure no one is happier this book is finally done than you!

The Biopolitical and Affective Dimensions of Beauty

I first heard the phrase "Não tem feio, só tem pobre" (There are no ugly people, only poor people) early in my fieldwork in southeastern Brazil, from my twenty-six-year-old black friend Samara, who was looking through a magazine profiling the latest trends in plastic surgery, called *Plástica e Beleza* (Plastic Surgery and Beauty). Samara viscerally hated the *nariz grosso* (thick nose) that she had been born with and was considering either saving up the money for a nose job at a private clinic or facing the long queue for a cheaper surgery at a public hospital. I was perplexed, because I had always thought Samara had an otherworldly beauty about her, with her androgynous look, high cheekbones, and strong eyebrows. Despite it being an early point in what turned out to be several years of friendship, I already admired Samara for her brilliant mind, for her eclectic tastes, and for the strength it took for her to come out as transgender to her parents and friends. She identified as nonbinary, and therefore she played with gender every day, pushing the boundaries of what masculinity and femininity were supposed to embody.

I told Samara that I did not think she needed a nose job, but she informed me that the social reality was that thinner noses, like the ones advertised as beautiful by light-skinned models in magazines, were clearly more desirable to everyone in Brazilian society. As Samara leafed through the magazine, she commented on the before and after pictures of celebrities profiled in the magazine—whose nose jobs had turned out well, and whose had not, or who looked ten years younger after a face-lift. Eventually, she closed the magazine with a sigh and exclaimed, "It's undeniably true: there are no ugly people, only poor people." The phrase implies that no one is ugly by choice, that ugly people are ugly only because they cannot afford to become beautiful through plastic surgery and other beautification techniques. Ugliness, in other words, is an unequivocal signifier of poverty, because wealth can immediately buy you beauty. Ugliness is not a biological destiny but a state of being that is subject to correction and improvement.

The phrase "There are no ugly people, only poor people" would recur time and again during my two years of fieldwork, uttered by a wide variety of interviewees in very different contexts. Surprisingly, it was not wealthy Brazilians from whom I heard that phrase most often but working-class interviewees, who interpreted beauty as a resource that had been denied to them. My friend Samara, for example, came from a poor family in rural São Paulo and now worked as a bank teller in the city. This position gave her a certain amount of economic stability, but it by no means made her affluent and she struggled to make ends meet. She identified as *pobre* (poor), a category that working-class Brazilians commonly use in contrast to those they identify as *ricos*—the wealthy.

When I asked Samara to elaborate on what she meant by the phrase she had used, she said, "I believe there are social classes where there are more beautiful people. I believe that the more money you have, the greater the probability that you are more beautiful. For various reasons: you eat better, you lead a better life, you can get plastic surgery. . . . Of course, there are beautiful poor people and very ugly rich people. But most rich people I see are beautiful, and when they are not naturally beautiful they *make* themselves beautiful." Samara fantasized on several occasions about all the surgeries she would have if she had unlimited money, and she lamented the limited opportunity she had to make beauty a reality for herself, as someone who was poor. Samara's reasoning was not unique—nearly all of my working-class interviewees in Brazil, no matter their color or gender identity, shared this understanding of beauty as closely correlating with wealth. They perceived their bodies as more prone to aging because they led harder lives and did not have the time or resources to continuously maintain their bodies. An unhealthy and troubled life is considered especially detrimental to a person's beauty, leaving that person *acabada* (finished, spent).

Beauty, I eventually came to understand, is closely associated with wealth because it is considered a form of capital that has real consequences for one's social standing. Working-class Brazilians firmly believe that having a *boa aparência* (good appearance) is essential in the job market, because if one's looks signify humble origins, there are few chances of getting a white-collar job that pays better than average. On the flip side, narratives of how beauty can provide upward mobility abound in Brazilian media—particularly in soap operas and reality-show beauty contests, where poor but light-skinned women are recognized for their beauty, either by a male lead or a modeling scout, and suddenly marry into a wealthier family, achieve fame, or are awarded a modeling contract.

These narratives are highly gendered—it is usually women who are considered upwardly mobile because of their beauty—but it is becoming increasingly common for men to be recognized for their beauty as well. A particularly striking case was *o mendigo gato* (the handsome beggar)— a thirty-year-old man who became famous after a woman posted on Facebook a picture of him begging for change in the streets of Curitiba, making him a viral sensation overnight. People were surprised that such a handsome man—with blue eyes, light skin, and European features— would be begging on the streets, and many sought to help him out financially and tried to reunite him with his family. Eventually, he was revealed to have fallen into poverty because of a drug addiction. The media followed him for months, chronicling his rehabilitation, his online fandom, and the launch of his modeling career (since many fashion lines immediately perceived the marketing opportunity he represented). His economic recovery seemed to be a self-fulfilling prophecy, destined by his appearance.

It seems ironic that thousands of darker-skinned people begging in the streets of Brazil go unrecognized every day; they are deemed to be where they belong because they do not possess the qualities that would provide them with the capital known as beauty. Beauty not only mimics the colorism of the Brazilian social hierarchy—in which being poor closely correlates with being darker skinned—but is also one of the central ways by which racialized characteristics acquire positive and negative value. I had another interesting conversation about beauty with my friend Samara a few years later, after she had begun to proudly identify as a black feminist, influenced by classes on race and gender that she had taken at college. Despite her newfound critical consciousness and her awareness that all aesthetic evaluations are social constructions, she struggled to embrace her own appearance and was still considering a nose job. She told me, "I know I am coopted by Caucasian beauty standards; it's shitty." There were days she simply felt ugly. She also struggled with the pressure to abandon her androgynous look and conform to a standard femininity, knowing well it would make her more attractive in the eyes of others.

Yet Samara also found immense pleasure in her daily beauty routines, such as putting on makeup, straightening her hair, and experimenting with different eyeshadows and hairstyles depending on the occasion. Part of her daily routine consisted in straightening her Afro-textured hair because it would otherwise be considered "unkempt" and inappropriate for her workplace. Making herself beautiful for a night on the town, however, was one of the central ways that Samara made herself matter and recognizable to others. To Samara, beauty was both a burden and a boon, something that she did not have the privilege to ignore or to simply analyze in academic fashion. As I watched her straighten and shape her hair before going out one night, I marveled at her talent for creating new, bold hairstyles, constantly refusing any illusion of fixity, even as she worked to alter her hair from its natural state because Brazilian society considered it "bad hair." Beauty is a biopolitical regime that people feel compelled to follow, but it is also a felt relation to one's own body as well as a form of becoming.

THE MAGICIANS OF BEAUTY

In this book, I argue that beauty matters in Brazil because it produces forms of affect that condense race, class, and gender inequalities onto and through the body, generating an aesthetic hierarchy that produces a scale of value ranging from the beautiful and normative to the ugly and abject. This aesthetic hierarchy is highly mobile, because beautification practices promise to revalue those whose bodies are deemed lower in the aesthetic hierarchy, even if it seems like a Sisyphean task, repeated endlessly. Most of my interviewees understood beautification not as a question of vanity but as a characteristic central to their social worth and to opportunities for social mobility. As the Brazilian popular saying asserts, "A beleza abre portas" (Beauty opens doors)—beauty gives a body social value and creates the conditions of possibility for human dignity and happiness. Ugliness, on the other hand, is experienced as a source of social exclusion and suffering.

For example, most of my working-class interviewees who actively sought plastic surgery expressed how ugliness had caused them suffering, and they believed that beautification would improve their lives. The standard of beauty was critiqued as unfair and unrealistic, and it was described as an oppressive system: many called this beauty ideal *a ditadura da beleza* (the dictatorship of beauty). At the same time, most felt that foregoing beauty altogether was not an option, because it would mean risking their worth in society. Beauty is fetishized as a good in itself, despite most people's understanding that, as a value, it arises from social relationships—one is "ugly" only in relation to more "beautiful" others, real or imagined, that one aspires to resemble (even if it is only an idealized version of oneself). Beauty can be understood as what Sara Ahmed calls a "relational object," insofar as it does not reside within any particular subject but becomes "saturated with affect" only as a product of its circulation.[1] It is this very relationality that makes beauty feel like a "dictatorship"—a system of social relations that imposes an aesthetic hierarchy and threatens those who dare disobey with social death.

I almost never heard a word of criticism, however, regarding *os magos da beleza* (the magicians of beauty), as plastic surgeons are frequently called. As purveyors of valuable capital, they are highly admired for their ability to reappraise bodies that are considered devalued, depreciated, or diminished. Stories abound in popular culture about "miracles" performed by plastic surgeons, such as the skin grafts on the racecar driver disfigured by burns, the salvaged ear on the businessman mutilated by his kidnappers, and the hair implants on the woman scalped by a motorboat propeller. Plastic surgeons themselves are experts at circulating those stories by promoting media coverage of specific instances of surgical heroism, despite their rarity compared to everyday aesthetic procedures.

In a society where structural violence seems to be a norm, plastic surgeons portray themselves as healers of the body and the body politic, providing everyone with the chance to be beautiful again. Working-class Brazilians, in particular, are thankful for the expansion of plastic surgery into the public health-care system in the last few decades, which means that plastic surgery is now accessible for free or at much lower prices than in the private clinics. Low-income patients vying for plastic surgery in the public health-care system expressed to me how thankful they were to the plastic surgeons who made this possible. It made them feel as if they, too, now had access to those miracles of beautification that were usually a privilege of the wealthy. Even patients whose surgeries had gone unexpectedly wrong (causing them a huge amount of distress) expressed anger only at the doctor who had made the mistake, not at the medical discipline in general, because they still had hope that another plastic surgeon, with more talent and skill than the previous one, would be able to correct the damage done.

One surgeon, in particular, stood above all others as the most admired plastic surgeon in Brazil: Ivo Pitanguy. An icon of Brazilian medicine, Pitanguy was a veritable celebrity until his passing in 2016, and he remains a household name. Back in the 1960s, Pitanguy was the first to propose that the poor, too, have the right to beauty and should not be excluded from plastic surgery. With the backing of then-president Juscelino Kubitschek, Pitanguy opened the first center that offered plastic surgery to low-income patients, at a philanthropic Catholic hospital called Santa Casa da Misericórdia, located in Rio de Janeiro. Even today, the Santa Casa is a symbol of Pitanguy's humanitarian concern for the poor and is in such high demand that prospective patients wait months or even years for the surgical procedures it offers.

Many of the patients I interviewed at Santa Casa specifically said that Pitanguy's reputation was what brought them there for surgery, despite the long wait (now that it is possible to get plastic surgery in many other hospitals in the public health-care system). For instance, Renata, a fifty-three-year-old working-class patient, expressed her utmost admiration for Pitanguy: "Ivo Pitanguy is a synonym of plastic surgery, he is the father, the god of plastic surgery. He is a god in Brazil, in the whole world, I believe. That is why the Santa Casa has credibility. He has operated on people who have had their entire bodies burned. He has also operated on many famous people. . . . But he is still simple, and has an immense wisdom." Renata's characterization of Pitanguy as an almost saintly figure—a veritable "god of plastic surgery"—was not unique. When I was doing research he was already in ill health and rarely frequented the Santa Casa, but patients yearned to catch a glimpse of him, hopeful that his presence would somehow guarantee that their surgery went well. Despite their commitment to surgery, patients were perfectly aware that the Santa Casa doubles as a medical school, and that medical residents still in training perform most of the surgeries. Risk was high, but faith in Pitanguy was higher.

Pitanguy is still revered in Brazil because he represented the pinnacle of the powers of plastic surgery. A Brazilian adage summarizes the skills with which he was imbued in the popular imagination: when someone or something is so unforgivably ugly that it is simply beyond repair, people may remark that "nem o Pitanguy da jeito" (not even Pitanguy could fix this). In normal circumstances, however, very little was considered beyond the power of Pitanguy's scalpel. All other surgeons try to borrow from the symbolic capital his image represents, and those who graduated from his medical school or from a school operated by one of his students boast of their connection to him, even if it is once or twice removed. This imagined lineage has real consequences for their ability to attract private clients and earn an income.

Even doctors from other medical specialties try to associate themselves with plastic surgery to gain the social capital and economic advantages associated with the beautification industry: dermatologists advertise skin-rejuvenating procedures, obstetricians specialize in tummy tucks along with C-sections, endocrinologists give out prescriptions for weight-loss pills, and gastroenterologists offer bariatric surgery as a form of weight control. The biopolitical injunction to be beautiful is backed by a powerful scientific discourse, but it is simultaneously permeated by magical thinking—the perception that the secret to eternal beauty is just around the corner. The magico-religious power attributed to plastic surgery is so great that beauty salons now advertise a specific type of hair straightening as *plástica para os cabelos* (plastic surgery for the hair), and a few evangelical churches promise rapid weight loss and *lipoaspiração divina* (divine lipo-suction) through special prayers. The magicians of beauty are everywhere, selling their wares to a public that is skeptical but also desperate to believe.

BEYOND AGENCY AND STRUCTURE

Ever since I began doing research on this project, I have been wary about portraying Brazilians as dupes of the beautification industry or as irra-tional actors who uncritically fall for the magic of beauty. I wanted to faithfully portray the critiques that arose organically from the embodied experiences of patients, even as I chronicled how they urgently tried to keep up with the demands of the beauty regimes they live in. Most anthropologists, sociologists, and cultural theorists who write about plastic surgery face this delicate balancing act, seeking to find agency in the desires of plastic surgery patients while still critiquing the ways in which plastic surgery reproduces a normative body that devalues forms of bodily difference.[2] The pitfall of this approach is that it remains caught in a structure-versus-agency paradox, where the agency of subjects arises only in response to the rigid social structures they face. In addition, this approach does not entirely explain either the visceral allure of beauty as a bodily quality or the faith people put in it.

For example, the literature on plastic surgery in Brazil has followed two distinct paths. On one hand, we have the work of Joana de Vilhena

Novaes, which critiques the medical discourse that associates thinness and fitness with beauty, and which portrays female patients as simply internalizing those patriarchal norms—there is little room for agency in her work, and no analysis of race.[3] On the other hand, we have the work of Mirian Goldenberg and Alexander Edmonds, who analyze plastic surgery in Brazil mainly as an expansion of consumption practices onto the body itself, and who are surprisingly uncritical of the scientific discourses that underlie this particular medical practice.[4] Edmonds explicitly critiques the Foucauldian approaches that "stress the function of biomedicine as a form of discipline and social control" by the state, proposing we instead understand beauty as a way for patients to aspire to modernity, and as a great social equalizer because it is surprisingly capable of challenging traditional hierarchies.[5]

All of these accounts of plastic surgery, however, largely ignore the longer history of beauty in Brazil and the extent to which the discourses of surgeons are informed by eugenic thought and by a desire to produce a racially homogenous population. Very early in my research, I realized that the expansion of plastic surgery into public hospitals was based on a particular biopolitical vision for the nation, which explicitly ranked some bodies as more desirable than others. Mimi Thi Nguyen warns us that beauty is not a politically neutral category but, rather, a form of biopower that instrumentalizes notions of empowerment to render certain bodies as legible and others as premodern, barbaric, or in need of liberation.[6] Beauty, in other words, produces forms of governmentality that manage the body in particular ways.

Influenced by a science and technology studies framework, I became interested in the ways that plastic surgeons, medical residents, and other health professionals justify beautification as a national project. Taking into account Bruno Latour's suggestion that we follow scientists "in action" as they craft networks, resolve controversies, and recruit allies for their practice,[7] I spent a significant portion of my research time interviewing doctors at their medical offices, at conferences they attended, in the hallways of hospitals and clinics, and even in the operating rooms where they supervised their medical students' surgical proficiency. I was fortunate that a couple of plastic surgeons who served as directors of three residency programs, two in Belo Horizonte and one in Rio de Janeiro, decided I would get a clearer sense of how they served low-income populations if I simply donned a lab coat or scrubs and followed them around several public hospitals that doubled as teaching hospitals. These two surgeons, and any medical staff I encountered, simply assumed that low-income patients were the obvious population for me to "study," because that population was also the one on which they built their own knowledge and carried out scientific studies. Even though I was careful to always reveal my identity as an anthropologist and ask for consent before I interviewed anyone, it surprised me how naturally patients took to my presence, knowing well that they were case studies for medical students who were also in their late twenties, as I was at the time.

Trying to avoid replicating the unequal power relations inherent in medical research, I sought to situate not only the discourses of patients but also the knowledge of plastic surgeons within the context in which they emerged. I carried out significant archival research in the Biblioteca Nacional (National Library) in Rio de Janeiro, tracing the ways in which narratives about race, gender, nation, and population had informed medical discourses about beauty in Brazil since the early twentieth century (see chapter 1). Although I acknowledge that these medical discourses have undergone important historical shifts over the last century, I also take into account Donna Haraway's assertion that "key objects of knowledge" such as race and population semiotically carry over certain patterns of power and authority into the present.[8]

The anthropological study of science, in addition, provided me with three key insights regarding the ways that science and society are coconstituted, revealing the messy complexities of producing scientific knowledge. First, scholars like Lesley Sharp and Elizabeth Roberts demonstrate that moral judgments are usually disavowed by scientific actors yet permeate their thinking[9]—which made me cognizant of how medical "facts" reveal the understated moral judgments plastic surgeons make about bodies and their worth. Second, many anthropologists have pointed out that experimental subjects are central to the development of scientific knowledge, but also how frequently that form of labor and capital becomes invisible[10]—leading me to recognize how plastic surgery relies on experimental subjects for its continuity. Finally, Emily Martin points out that despite the appearance of science as an impenetrable citadel, we can, as anthropologists, track the underlying rhizomic connections between scientific institutions, private interests, the public, and the state that make science possible in the first place.[11] I found that, owing to the weakness of the Brazilian government, plastic surgeons become the de facto representatives of the state in public hospitals, enforcing a form of neoliberal governmentality that benefits their private interests as well (see chapter 2). We cannot, therefore, afford to ignore how plastic surgery intersects with the state in Brazil, as most of the scholarship on plastic surgery in Brazil has done.

Alexander Edmonds has a point, however, when he warns us against relying too much on Foucault to explain the appeal of beauty. One of the surprising aspects of my interviews and conversations with patients was how little overlap I found between their conceptions of why beauty mattered and the medical discourse of plastic surgeons. To say that patients simply internalized medical norms would be to miss the ways in which patients related their desire for beauty to the gender, class, and race inequalities they faced every day—they had embodied responses to beauty's perceived scarcity. As Elizabeth Grosz argues, the Foucauldian portrayal of the body as an inscriptive surface, on which disciplinary regimes are imposed and through which discursive power is mobilized, presents the body as problematically passive.[12]

Judith Butler complicated Foucault's account by portraying bodies as materializing through the constant reiteration of norms and regulatory schemas, producing the semblance of fixity over time. She argues that "sex is both produced and destabilized in the course of this reiteration," because any instance of replicating gender norms also produces new openings for gender performances that exceed the norm, resignifying and transforming gender in the process.[13] Anthropologists who study gender, however, are skeptical that this process of resignification works on the ground. Saba Mahmood makes the case that Muslim women in Egypt neither consolidate nor subvert gender norms through their performances of piety, but rather inhabit and consummate norms in surprising ways.[14] Similarly, Ann Marie Leshkowich argues that Vietnamese women who adopt essentialist notions of gender are nonetheless able to produce social change by asserting their gendered subjectivity in a context of economic transformation.[15] According to Margot Weiss, even gender and sexual practices that seem transgressive, like BDSM in San Francisco, rely on the ambivalent embodiment of social norms to produce sexual desire, in ways that complicate the reiteration/resignification binary.[16] Thus, Butler's schema falls short because it misses the ways in which embodiment is a lived, corporeal response to changing social milieus, and not simply a reiteration of norms and discourses.

Following Marcia Ochoa's critique of Butler,[17] we can argue that as much as Butler insists on the materiality of the body, she nonetheless reduces the messiness and carnality of the flesh to the logocentric embodiment of signs. In Butler's conception, the body is not an entity that bleeds, leaks, or, in Diane Nelson's word, "splatters" as it encounters the violence of biopolitical norms.[18] Returning briefly to Mahmood, we have to account for the ways in which our interviewees "treat the body as a medium for, rather than a sign of, the self. . . . [W]hat is required is a much deeper engagement with the architecture of the self that undergirds a particular mode of living and attachment."[19] In my own research, this deeper engagement with the architecture of the self has meant paying attention to embodied forms of perception and cognition that seem to reside beyond, or to precede, language.

If beauty is not simply a straightforward materialization of biopolitical discourses, how do we explain why beauty is felt so viscerally by subjects, as an evaluation of oneself or another that occurs nearly instantaneously and below the level of awareness? Alexander Edmonds resorts to biologizing beauty, arguing that perhaps we have been missing a "biological stratum of experience" that explains why beauty engages us in particular ways.[20] I am wary, however, of any universalizing account that does not see beauty as emerging from accumulated layers of historical and cultural patterns that give meaning to the body. Instead, I look to the literature on affect to understand perceptions of beauty as gut reactions that are entirely social, but which are not subject to modification, at least not with ease, because they have become habitual at a preconscious level. I find affect conceptually useful because it allows us to consider an even earlier moment in the process of socialization, one in which perception itself emerges as an embodied response to social relationships.[21] In the words of William Mazzarella, affect gets at the ways in which "society is inscribed in our nervous system and in our flesh before it appears in our consciousness."[22]

Conceiving perception itself as a social interface allows us to imagine the body as emerging from the world it interacts with, not as simply docile or resistant to power structures. Thus, we come to understand embodiment not as predetermined by discourse but rather as an unpredictable process of sociality. I am particularly inspired by Sara Ahmed's description of how affect circulates through the body politic and sticks to or accumulates on certain bodies or body parts, imparting positive or negative value at the very level of perception.[23] For example, how is it that Samara's wider nose came to be considered an "ugly" trait in Brazil? Such aesthetic evaluation cannot be divorced from a long history of racism that devalues black facial characteristics; nonetheless, this aesthetic evaluation has become second nature for a majority of Brazilians—they simply perceive wider noses as aesthetically unattractive.

Nonetheless, while surgeons (nearly all of them light-skinned) naturalized the inferiority of what they called the "negroid nose" through medical discourse (see chapter 5), working-class, darker-skinned Brazilians related their desire for a nose job directly to racial prejudice and to unequal opportunities in the workplace (see chapter 3). For both, the nose is a site of affective investment, yet the same bodily appendage enables different forms of "racial mattering," to use Mel Chen's terminology.[24] Embodied experiences, in other words, allow working-class patients to perceive the same surgical events differently than their surgeons do. These patients' very perceptions of beauty are transforming beauty into an arena of struggle, where the threat of abjection is always present, but also where there is simultaneously a potential for beauty to be redefined beyond the constraints of discourse. Like Samara's constant change of hairstyle after straightening her hair, our perceptions of beauty always exceed our words for it.

Moreover, while the biopolitical discourses of surgeons always reduce beauty to the visual realm (obsessed as they are with photography and anthropometry), affect accounts for the ways in which beauty inhabits the other senses. Few people can convey exactly what they find physically attractive in another human being, aside from appearance, and yet the ineffable forms of beauty are central to its sway over us. Perhaps it is something about a person's scent in the morning, the way someone's presence engages a room, the timbre of someone's voice, or the texture of that person's lips. A perception of beauty in another triggers individual memories, emotions, and other embodied experiences: the perception reminds the beholder of other people he or she has loved, desired, or admired, and it is also reminiscent of abstract qualities like style, charisma, wit, strength, or congeniality.

Additionally, each perception of beauty in another has a dynamic relationship with one's own self-perception and one's lived experience within the human body—a body that is always changing, never in stasis—which means one's tastes change as one's body ages. Even though these perceptual experiences might seem natural, nearly visceral, to an individual, they are embedded in a longer history and a social context that give meaning to the senses beyond the individual. One learns to "see" and "feel" beauty in the same way one learns other behaviors and habits: by living in and participating in a community that shares experiences and knowledge. Affect theory holds that perceptions are forged through the sensory interface between individuals and their surroundings: the senses would remain numb if they remained isolated from interaction.[25] In order to understand beauty anthropologically, therefore, we must rethink embodied perception as mediated through our ability to inhabit spaces, people, and objects beyond ourselves.

Instead of framing biopolitical discourse as a kind of structure that patients either submit to or actively resist, we should understand biopolitical discourse and sensory perception as mutually constitutive forces animated by affect that refract and feed off each other during the constitution of the subject. As Patricia Clough argues, the affective turn is attuned to the materiality and dynamism of the body as it engages with the biopolitical discourses it encounters: "What is important now in returning to Foucault's argument about biopolitics is that there is a new fold in its fabric[:] . . . the meshing of politics, of biopolitics, with an economy of affect."[26] Affect, I believe, provides a better explanation for why power extends so efficiently throughout society, through mechanisms that Foucault simply described as capillary and micropolitical, but which he did not engage any further. Affect also explains why resistance is already embedded in our compliance with power—we are affectively attuned to power, providing it the intensity it needs to exist in the first place, but our perceptions are not entirely defined by the ways power crystallizes into certain patterns, because we all have different experiences of embodiment.[27]

I disagree with the critique of affect theory that claims it has a proclivity to evacuate the subject and to lose the social context in which intentionality can occur and, thus, contradicts the ethnographic attention to agency.[28] Ethnography has long regarded forms of embodiment as windows to subject formation,[29] but affect adds a particular insight into the socialization of our very perceptions, and connects this socialization to the intersubjective processes that occur beyond the subject as well—it adds layers to the complexities of subject formation rather than evacuates subjectivity. Anthropology, in fact, is probably uniquely positioned to intervene in affect theory by demonstrating that historical and cultural context are central to the emergence of our embodied perceptions, providing a counterpoint to the few theorists who rely too much on universalist neuroscientific claims about personhood to understand affect.[30]

AFFECTIVE CAPITAL

The affective and biopolitical dimensions of beauty in Brazil are inextricable from capitalism and its ability to assign value to the body in particular ways. Beauty is a key aspect of sociality in Brazil because it immediately communicates a body's social standing—its relative worth in relation to other bodies. For example, people use the phrase *gente bonita* (beautiful people) as a euphemism for people who are lighter skinned and who exhibit the trappings of wealth. An up-and-coming locale, for instance, is valued not according to its price of admission or its fare but, rather, according to the amount of *gente bonita* who frequent it. In contrast, I frequently heard the phrase *pobre, preto, e feio* (poor, black, and ugly), usually in the context of a crude joke, to describe the perfect trifecta of undesirability—the abject other to social worth. The physical features that are undesirable also mark certain bodies as racially and economically inferior in the rigid Brazilian social hierarchy, undeserving of social recognition and full citizenship within the nation.

Since the body is considered to be infinitely malleable,[31] however, individuals who climb the social ladder are expected to transform their bodies to conform to upper-class standards. Those with the resources and time to become beautiful, the logic goes, will undoubtedly do so. My interviewees explained to me that the first thing people do upon becoming successful is to straighten their hair and get thinner noses via plastic surgery. Beautification practices, especially plastic surgery, are valued so highly because they claim the power to produce value out of ugliness, which seems like the alchemist's ability to transmute lead into gold. Plastic surgeons are perfectly aware of this and market their techniques as instant bodily transformations reminiscent of fairy tales.

As several anthropologists have noted, magical thinking is becoming a common characteristic of late capitalism because the economic promise of upward mobility is fragile and precarious, leading people to put their faith in noneconomic means of advancement.[32] Social hierarchies in Brazil remain remarkably rigid, despite more than a decade of rule by the center-left Workers' Party, which made significant progress toward reducing extreme poverty but did not dismantle the power structures in place. Despite celebratory claims about the emergence of a "new middle class," for example, most of the new jobs that these Brazilians occupied were still working-class positions with little or no promise of further advancement.[33] The measurable increase in the purchasing power of the working class did not translate into changes to the overall economic pyramid, and the new neoliberal government that was forcibly installed in 2016 is slowly dismantling the safety net that had marginally protected the working class.

At the time my research took place, any new consumers who were created during Brazil's brief economic boom seemed to be increasingly putting their faith in beautification as a way to reaffirm the small socioeconomic gains they had made. The beauty and hygiene sector of the

Brazilian economy has had real growth, adjusted for inflation, of more than 100 percent since the year 2000, mostly owing to an explosion in the consumption of beauty and hygiene products among low-income Brazilians.[34] Even during the recent severe economic crisis, the beauty and hygiene sector grew a surprising 7 percent, seemingly immune to the contraction of the GDP.[35] Brazil is now the world's third-largest consumer of beauty and hygiene products, trailing behind only China and the United States, and the second-largest consumer of plastic surgery.[36] These numbers are outstanding, given the size of the Brazilian economy. The national preoccupation with beauty cannot be reduced to a straightforward consumer boom or an individualistic search for self-esteem. Beauty is, above all, a set of social relations that arrange the body politic in a particular manner.

The strong element of magical thinking that is linked with beautification should be understood within a larger context: the unnatural qualities of capitalism and the hierarchies it produces. As Michael Taussig argues, there is nothing natural about the accumulation of capital itself. The fact that money can be invested to produce new capital, in the form of interest, was interpreted by the Colombian peasants he interviewed in the 1970s as a form of dark magic or a pact with the devil. Taussig reverses the anthropological gaze on our society, to demonstrate that from the point of view of those who have not yet internalized the accumulation of profit as natural, capitalism is as magical an operation as any other and, perhaps, more sinister.[37] He believed that the peasants contested the fetishization of money as a value in itself because the peasant's gift-economy conceived of all things as embedded in relational networks, and comprehended that "things interact because of meanings they carry—sensuous, interactive, animate meanings of transitiveness."[38]

When Taussig returned to the same region of Colombia forty years later, however, he discovered that even poor people were now invested in a new form of magic: the seemingly endless power of beautification and plastic surgery to transform the human body. The value of work had been replaced with the value of fashion, style, and consumption, with the body as the ultimate commodity to be enhanced.[39] Despite Taussig's failure to fully historicize the race, class, and gender dynamics that shape plastic surgery practices in Colombia, what I find compelling about Taussig revisiting his old fieldsite is his realization that the magical thinking that he had once felt was an element of the peasants' latent critique of capitalism now allows the beauty industry to flourish. Those same "sensuous, interactive, animate meanings of transitiveness" that once helped to denaturalize capitalism now imbue all social relations with economic value, even the body itself. The transitive properties of affect, in other words, have been integrated into the economy as immaterial forms of value.

Late capitalism thrives on this new immaterial economy that emphasizes image and surface over content and monetizes forms of affect and emotion.[40] There is no longer an outside to capitalistic logic, and capitalism thrives on the magical thinking promoted by advertising, which seeks to craft associations between consumption and the most intimate aspects of our lives and identities. Acknowledging that forms of embodiment have become immaterial forms of value, however, means that we should reconsider the ways through which affective qualities such as beauty become fetishized as values in themselves. Sara Ahmed has pointed out that affect is akin to capital, insofar as it is only through the circulation of affect that it becomes aligned with specific bodies and communities, and it is only through its movement that some signs increase in affective value over time.[41] I wish to extend her argument by making the case that the affective economy produced by beauty functions particularly well in late capitalism because it produces value through the movement of bodies upward or downward in Brazil's aesthetic hierarchy, in the same way that commodities produce surplus value through their circulation in the marketplace.

In other words, the affect tied to beauty is not only comparable to capital, but it also produces its own parallel form of *affective capital* that is then imagined as convertible into economic capital, and vice versa, accompanying the movement of a person's place in Brazilian society. My interviewees' insistence that beautification was not simply a form of vanity, that it had real effects on their social and economic standing, reflects this equivalence between beauty, as a form of affective capital, and the more tangible economic capital. Refusing to participate in the affective economy produced by beauty is just as implausible as refusing to participate in the labor economy—both money and beauty are essential aspects of having worth in society, and they are understood as buttressing each other in fundamental ways. Ugliness *is* a form of poverty.

The type of capital that I am describing is akin to what Pierre Bourdieu calls "cultural capital"—a set of bodily dispositions carefully cultivated to legitimize one's position within a social hierarchy. Cultural capital is highly naturalized, becoming indistinguishable from the person who carries it—in fact, it gives that person value over others. It also gives that person clear economic advantages over others in areas such as the job market and the marriage marketplace.[42] Bourdieu, however, imagines the very value of cultural capital as arising from a relatively stable classification system that opposes the refined and distinguished tastes of the dominant class to the vulgar or ordinary preferences of the masses. In other words, cultural capital is largely inaccessible to those without power in society, who, by embracing the uncultured tastes attributed to them, end up "condemning themselves to what is in any case their lot."[43]

Not only have insights from cultural studies complicated this portrayal of how the reception of popular culture works in practice,[44] but also Bourdieu mistakenly assumes that the aesthetic preferences of the working class and the upper class are always in opposition to one another. Thus, despite being cognizant of the ways in which beauty is cultivated by women of the dominant classes, Bourdieu, when confronted with the "fact" that beauty is sometimes present among the economically unprivileged as well, resorts to biologizing beauty as an effect of "social heredity" that potentially "threatens the other social hierarchies" produced by cultural capital.[45] The literature that has examined beauty in Brazil follows Bourdieu and interprets beauty either as a form of bodily capital imposed by the dominant class and then imitated by the rest of society, or as a "democratizing" biological force that can upend the existing social hierarchies.[46]

By deploying the notion of affective capital, I attempt to complicate these explanations of why beauty matters in Brazil, by providing a more complex picture of how beauty is produced, communicated, and reinterpreted. First, I do not regard notions of beauty as being produced at the top and then trickling down to the rest of society. As an affective quality and a form of biopower, beauty permeates the social landscape and does not have a specific location; nor does one particular social class have a monopoly on its meanings. During my fieldwork, I was surprised to find that the fear of being perceived as ugly exists even among the most privileged members of Brazilian society, who submit their bodies to surgical corrections for even the tiniest imperfections that distance them from whiteness or gender normativity.

Second, beauty produces value because it promises to make bodies circulate within the existing aesthetic hierarchy—it continuously generates an illusion of upward mobility among those who are recognized as beautiful and renders everyone's position within the body politic as permanently precarious, a single misstep away from social exclusion. Beauty does not democratize Brazilian society but, rather, reaffirms the notion that some body types and facial characteristics have more value than others, no matter where these bodies are located in society.

Last, and most important, beauty is a form of capital that strongly relies on the transitive properties of affect—the transference of the meanings attributed to one set of relationships (race, class, and gender hierarchies) to a second set of relationships (beauty and ugliness). These associations are not haphazard—they are the product of a biopolitical history that prescribes which bodies conform to national ideals and are to be emulated, and which are deviant or dangerous. These associations affectively emerge from a social milieu that considers certain bodies as socially and economically valuable and, therefore, as bodies that enable upward mobility to a lucky few, producing hope and "promising happiness" to those invested in performances of beauty (see chapter 4).[47]

I am not the first scholar to use the term *affective capital* for the Brazilian context. In her fantastic ethnography *The Color of Love*, the sociologist Elizabeth Hordge-Freeman describes the damaging effects of racism within Brazilian families, where darker-skinned or otherwise racially marked individuals are considered ugly, are treated with disdain, and are provided fewer opportunities by their own family members, particularly their parents. She argues that possessing devalued racial features reduces an individual's access to affective capital because it "leads to differential experiences of support, love and encouragement, which has a lasting impact on one's life chances."[48] Although we use the word *affective* in different ways—Hordge-Freeman uses the term to signal a sentiment and does not engage the wider literature on affect—we both identify white beauty as a form of embodied capital, and we both describe Brazil as having a clear "aesthetic hierarchy" that is inescapable for social actors. The fact that we both, independently of each other, developed similar frameworks to talk about beauty and race in Brazil indicates the importance of beauty's role in the country's subtle but pervasive racial inequalities.

I hope that our work, read together, will provide a turning point in the scholarship about race in Brazil, which has long suggested that aesthetic evaluations are central to daily experiences of racism,[49] but which has not fully examined beauty as a social category—why beauty matters to Brazilians, how the national project of beautification is tied to eugenics, and how beauty allows for complex intersections between race, class, and gender inequality. The affective capital that is produced by beauty has very real material effects, facilitating the reproduction of the economic inequalities suffered by dark-skinned men and women, because it limits their work opportunities, their marriage prospects, their familial resources, and even their hopes of achieving any form of upward mobility.

A NOTE ON METHOD, POSITIONALITY, AND THE USE OF PSEUDONYMS

In this book I combine ethnographic fieldwork, archival research, and readings of popular culture in order to examine the prevailing notions of beauty in Brazil. I carried out this research over three nonconsecutive years: a main stretch of fieldwork between 2006 and 2008, and a second, less intensive one, between 2009 and 2011. Most of my ethnographic observations took place in Rio de Janeiro, considered the cultural capital of Brazil owing to its potent influence on national art, fashion, music, and literature, and given that it is where the largest media corporations, like Globo, are located. Its famous "beach culture" is undoubtedly prominent in people's self-definition, and some social scientists have said this explains the constant concern with beauty and fitness expressed by *cariocas,* as Rio de Janeiro residents are known.[50] To gauge whether plastic surgery is important to Brazilians who live farther away from the beach, I decided to also carry out ethnographic research in Belo Horizonte, the third-largest metropolitan region in Brazil and the capital of Minas Gerais, which neighbors the state of Rio de Janeiro. The ethnic composition of the two cities is similar: in both Rio de Janeiro and Belo Horizonte, about half the population identifies as white, and the other half identifies as black or brown.[51]

Comparing the two cities, I found that the residents of Belo Horizonte were as invested in beautification practices as *cariocas,* and that in both cities there were similar contrasts between working-class understandings of beauty and upper- or middle-class understandings of beauty. The biopolitical discourses of plastic surgeons in both locations were also very similar, tied as they were by a common lineage to Ivo Pitanguy's school of plastic surgery. I do not claim that these two southeastern Brazilian cities represent the country as a whole, or that interpretations of beauty do not differ in other regions. Nonetheless, most of the historical and contemporary representations of beauty in popular culture that I analyze have circulated nationwide, and I believe they have generated a national concern with beauty, even if regional specificities shape the way these messages about beauty are received.[52]

Most of my ethnographic research took place in teaching hospitals, always conducted with the permission of the hospital's chief plastic surgeon. As I mentioned earlier, in most cases I was treated like a new medical resident, which meant I was allowed to see the medical consultations, the psychological evaluations, and even the surgeries taking place on any given day. These events, however, revealed the biopolitical operations of plastic surgery more than the patients' motivations for surgery. The place where I preferred talking with patients was the waiting room, the only space where I was not required to wear a doctor's lab coat or scrubs and, thus, could mingle with patients more easily. The waiting room was usually full of lively conversations, since patients had to wait their turn for hours and were eager to exchange information with each other about how other patients' surgeries had gone and what to expect from the process. Most were happy to indulge my questions after I explained to them the nature of my research. I also had long conversations with patients and their family members in their hospital rooms as they recovered from surgery. About 90 percent of patients were female, and nearly all had a working-class background: they typically had working-class occupations and lived in low-income neighborhoods.

I complemented this research in the hospitals with informal interviews carried out in the neighborhood of São Gonçalo, a working-class district located inland in Rio de Janeiro state, about an hour's distance from the city's famous beaches. Over my three years of fieldwork, I visited this location almost every weekend with my roommate, Carlos, who had grown up there. I was particularly welcomed by his large extended family, which was incredibly hospitable and quickly began to treat me almost like a member of the family. I attended a wedding and a christening with this family, and I witnessed them struggle with the divorce of one family member and the death of another. It was through these ongoing relationships in São Gonçalo, sharing in these people's joys and sorrows, that I gained some of the greatest insights into what beauty meant to the Brazilian working class.

I had to develop a completely different approach in order to interview upper- and middle-class Brazilians. While plastic surgeons were entirely comfortable with my presence in teaching hospitals, assuming those patients were appropriate objects of study for me, only one surgeon was willing to let me approach his clients from his private practice. Surgeons wanted to protect the privacy of their wealthier clients and were perhaps worried that my probing questions might lose them a client. Thus, most of my interviews with upper- and middle-class patients were arranged through snowball sampling, by beginning with contacts I arranged through a local academic, and then by asking every interviewee to provide the names and contact information of friends who might want to be interviewed as well. These in-depth interviews took place in public locations, like cafes, bookstores, and malls, or within the private homes of patients.

Despite how forthcoming the upper- and middle-class patients I interviewed were, the fact that my research was structured by plastic surgeons meant I ended up with a much smaller sample of these patients compared to working-class patients. In total, I interviewed 24 upper- and middle-class patients and 173 working-class individuals over the course of my three years of fieldwork. The interviews with health professionals occurred organically as I spent time with them in the teaching hospitals, chatted with them in their offices, or attended medical conferences addressing beauty. I interviewed 71 health professionals in total, of which 8 were medical residents, 43 were plastic surgeons, 8 were medical staff who worked in private beauty clinics, and 12 were doctors from other medical specialties that were nonetheless invested in beautification. Finally, since narratives about poor women being discovered and turned into models abound in popular culture, I decided to carry out a few interviews in small modeling schools that were operating in two favelas, Cidade de Deus and Rocinha, and in a talent agency for children and teenagers located in Rio de Janeiro.

Ethnographic fieldwork is, in many ways, shaped by one's position in relation to one's subject matter. Anthropology has long since abandoned the veneer of objectivity, the idea that one's "informants" are completely knowable and that cultural patterns are transparent to anyone who looks hard enough. We are aware of the ways our discipline artificially constructs "ethnographic authority," and that knowledge, no matter its quality, is always partial and situated within a particular place and time.[53] We are also aware that interviewees shape what we see and respond in different ways to different anthropologists depending on our own subjectivity.

I did not expect, for example, that race would be such a central topic of my research—I initially became fascinated by plastic surgery because I was interested in issues of embodiment, gender, and medicalization. Plastic surgeons, however, could not seem to avoid the topic of race while in my presence and brought up it with such frequency that it became hard for me to ignore. Looking back, I suspect that surgeons identified me as an ally because I am Ecuadorian but very light-skinned, and because I seemed to be of a privileged background since I had acquired all my higher education in the United States. All plastic surgeons I interviewed belonged to the Brazilian elite, and all of them, except one (who was of Lebanese heritage), were very light-skinned. Surgeons would regularly make references to how "miscegenation" in Ecuador must be similar to that in Brazil, and to the fact that I, thus, should understand which racial mixtures made people beautiful. Many other light-skinned South Americans, most of them from wealthy backgrounds, were medical residents in the teaching hospitals where I carried out research—since Brazil is the ideal place to learn plastic surgery in the region—so my presence seemed to place me in a similar category. Perhaps it was how my subjectivity was read by plastic surgeons that enabled me to gain ready access to the spaces and the controversial musings of plastic surgeons.

My gender, too, very likely influenced what I was permitted to see. At all the teaching hospitals where I conducted research, all the plastic surgeons were male, and very few of the medical residents were female. Plastic surgery is still a male-dominated field in Brazil, and surgeons have a certain male camaraderie with one another that they happily extended to me. It was common, for example, for male surgeons to comment on the attractiveness of their female patients, and one explained to me that he used casual flirting to put his female patients at ease. What made me the most uncomfortable was the surgeons' assumption that they could ask working-class female patients to disrobe for examination in front me. It was usually I who stepped in and stopped the patient, asking her if she wanted me to leave the room first. Many female patients insisted I stay, saying they were used to being looked at by doctors, and that a medical anthropologist was no different—they seemingly considered me part of the male clinical gaze they expected at a teaching hospital, such as the photographs that surgeons rely on to measure the success of the surgery (see fig. 1).

In the case of working-class male patients, however, the surgeon would usually be more sensitive to the patient's privacy and ask me to leave the room during a medical examination. Male patients were in general much more reserved and unwilling to share with me their reasons for having surgery. As I explain more fully in chapter 3, plastic surgery is very much considered a feminine bodily practice, and men who opt for plastic surgery are stigmatized, unless it is a type of surgery designed to remasculinize the body. On a few but telling occasions, surgeons and other medical staff actively sought to disqualify patients perceived as gay or transgender from getting access to surgery and made homophobic or transphobic comments behind the patients' backs.

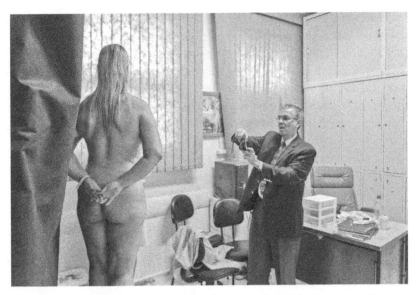

FIG 1. A plastic surgeon photographing a working-class patient before surgery. Photo courtesy of Vincent Rosenblatt.

Given this atmosphere, I never came out as gay to any of the health professionals I interviewed. I kept that part of my identity private lest it affect the rapport I had built with the people I was interviewing.[54]

I never challenged surgeons directly on their views or their practices, because I felt it was not my place to do so and it would have curtailed our conversations. I considered it my job as an ethnographer to take careful notes and be mindful of the milieu in which these medical tenets emerged and gained traction. I understand the worldview of plastic surgeons, as much as that of any other social group, as being shaped by their background, their privilege, and their collective beliefs, and I think most of them strove to make ethical decisions within the contingencies of their practice and the cultural context they were immersed in. My critiques of plastic surgery are not meant as critiques of the individual plastic surgeons I met with, who were generous with their time and were genuinely helpful in giving me access; instead, I wish to portray their concerns here as well. The unfettered expansion of plastic surgery is an issue that troubles these surgeons, because it devalues their practice and makes profit its only concern. My aim is to point out the race, class, and gender ideologies that underlie this expansion and how it compounds systemic problems already present in Brazilian health care.

For example, as I demonstrate in chapter 2, most teaching hospitals label aesthetic surgeries as reconstructive surgeries to get the public health care system to cover the costs, which means public resources are being redirected in problematic ways. In the same way that I use pseudonyms for all patients I interviewed, I have changed the names of all health professionals I interviewed and the names of hospitals and clinics where I carried out my research, because I do not want individual surgeons or institutions to be disciplined for a problem that is clearly systemic. The exceptions are the Santa Casa da Misericórdia and its iconic founder, Ivo Pitanguy, whose names I did not change because of their importance within the national imaginary and because the Santa Casa operates with funding donated by the association of Pitanguy's alums and, thus, avoids the use of public funding for these surgeries.

The contemporary photographs of patients and doctors that I have included on the cover and within this book are part of a photo essay titled *Plastic Surgery for the People* and were taken by Vincent Rosenblatt, a professional photographer who works in Brazil. These photographs do not depict any of my interviewees; and aside from those taken at the Santa Casa da Misericórdia, they focus on public hospitals other than the ones where I conducted research. I do not consider these photographs to be additional forms of ethnographic evidence, because as mediated texts these images were staged in particular ways and so are not straightforward representations of what I saw in the field. I included them nonetheless in order to present the reader with visual elements that contrast with the sanitized way that plastic surgery portrays itself in the public sphere—as a seamless transformation of the body, personified by idealized "before" and "after" pictures that rarely display the messy in-between.

The images from the photo essay can be read as a critical reflection on how every step of the process is marked by the medical gaze, from the markings and cuts that plastic surgeons make on the body to the depersonalization of the body on the operating table. The photographs also hint at the anticipation, anxiety, hope, and other forms of affect that mark the doctor-patient relationship. As João Biehl argues, photographs can be interesting companions to the work of ethnography, creating a different register through which to reflect on the partiality of any narrative. All we can present through either medium are the fragments of other people's lives, but these fragments matter, particularly when we portray people who normally go unheard.[55]

OUTLINE OF THE BOOK

In the chapters that follow, I combine two distinct theoretical approaches, Foucauldian biopolitics and affect theory, to explain the individual and collective forms of attachment to biotechnologies such as plastic surgery. I make the case that the popularization of plastic surgery arises from a mutually constitutive relationship between embodied, sensory relationships to medicine, and the biopolitical rationalities and forms of governance that embed doctors, patients, and the state in networks of knowledge and practice. I move back and forth between biopolitics and affect because this demonstrates the strength of each approach—while a Foucauldian approach is particularly useful in understanding the rise of beauty as a national project, I turn to affect theory to explain why patients find meaning in beauty and how beauty produces forms of affective capital that promise the movement of bodies within Brazil's aesthetic hierarchy. Biopolitical discourses are not simply inscribed on the bodies they intervene upon but are refracted through distinctive histories that produce new affective attachments regarding the bodies in question. In turn, these affective attachments feed into the forms of governance that shape how biotechnologies operate, grow, and transform across time and space, producing new subjectivities and new forms of capital. I hope to demonstrate that affect and biopolitics are impossible to disentangle from one another in the constitution of medicalized subjectivities, particularly under late capitalism.

Chapters 1 and 2 delineate the biopolitical framework that transformed beauty into a technology of biopower in Brazil. In the first chapter, which is based on archival research, I demonstrate that beauty developed as a central concern for the Brazilian eugenics movement in the early twentieth century as it became associated with improved hygienic practices and ongoing racial mixture, which eugenicists believed would inevitably whiten the nation as whole. The beauty of women—as the imagined bearers of future generations and as the objects of (male) medical scrutiny—was of particular concern. In other words, female beauty came to be understood as a symbol of the nation's progress, and beautification practices such as plastic surgery were lauded as sensible hygienic practices that aided the work of miscegenation.

Chapter 2 combines archival and ethnographic research to describe how Ivo Pitanguy, the main architect of the notion of the "right to beauty," borrowed from eugenic ideas to gain the support of the Brazilian state in the 1960s and open a medical school that would double as a plastic surgery service in a publicly funded hospital. This model of schooling for plastic surgeons has expanded widely, gaining nationwide recognition for plastic surgeons as humanitarians who care for the poor. I show that the Brazilian state is only marginally involved in this expansion of plastic surgery, because surgeons and residents borrow from the state's authority by deciding, within the confines of consultation rooms and operating rooms, which surgeries are approved and prioritized. What I call plastic governmentality elucidates how the state can become instrumentalized in the service of private interests under neoliberalism, by producing a pliable form of statecraft that uses statistics and medical discourse to gain support for cosmetic surgery while rendering biopolitically invisible those medical needs that are deemed unprofitable.

In chapters 3 and 4, I turn to the affective dimensions of beauty and beautification practices. The third chapter, which is based on ethnographic interviews with Brazilian patients, discusses the ways in which beauty makes bodies matter. I understand beauty as an affective quality that is not located in particular bodies, and that produces value only as it circulates between and through bodies, generating an aesthetic hierarchy that defines who matters in Brazilian society. This aesthetic hierarchy values gender normative bodies and renders women's bodies as more operable than male bodies. It also traffics in a form of racialized affect that values bodily characteristics associated with whiteness. However, working-class Brazilians have a complex affective relationship with beauty that tells a more complicated story of how their class, race, and gender come into being through beauty.

Chapter 4 examines the narratives of upward mobility through beauty that are interwoven throughout diverse forms of Brazilian media—from journalistic accounts of recently discovered models to the carefully crafted storylines of soap operas and televised beauty pageants. I compare these accounts from the media with ethnographic research among working-class parents who send their daughters to talent agencies or modeling schools. I argue that these girls' parents and teachers pin their hopes on performances of beauty because they understand the female body itself as a form of capital that promises a better future. This affective promise of a better future, however, becomes a moral injunction as well, sexualizing and racializing, in very particular ways, the poor women who are said to deserve upward mobility, emphasizing virtuous sexual behavior, European features, and straighter hair as essential components for success. I end the chapter by looking at an alternative beauty contest organized in Rio de Janeiro that challenges the moralism implicit in beauty, short-circuiting hope, and its emphasis on futurity.

The final two chapters make the case that the affective and biopolitical aspects of beauty combine in powerful ways to produce individual and collective investments in beauty as a national project. Chapter 5 addresses the racial logic that underpins the contemporary construction of beauty as a national health concern. Plastic surgeons portray their work as complementing the work of Brazilian miscegenation by correcting mistakes resulting from racial mixture. These corrections, however, always presume a higher desirability for whiter facial features, based on an aesthetic hierarchy that devalues and medicalizes non-European features, such as the diagnosable "negroid nose." This raciology of beauty, however, also relies on more diffuse forms of racialized affect, which blur the boundaries between bodies and thus produce whiteness as a fragile quality, as demonstrated by upper- and middle-class patients who seek beauty in order to differentiate themselves from the black body of the mulatta.

Chapter 6 analyzes the affective and biopolitical structures that produce low-income patients as willing experimental subjects. The chapter argues that the experimental settings of plastic surgery create medical and legal rationalities that externalize the risks of surgery onto the bodies of patients, diminishing the risks assumed by surgeons. Patients become entangled in the affective promises of surgery and make embodied, situated decisions that complicate our notions of medical consent. Surgeons can become attached to medical technologies that are riskier, because they promise them more control over the body, demonstrating that the neoliberal narrative of rational choice is insufficient to understand how decision making occurs within this medical context.

The conclusion reflects on the transnational dimensions of beauty. Beautification can be thought of as a global industry that takes on very different registers depending on the specific histories and the body politics where it emerges. Nonetheless, there are common methodologies and theoretical insights that allow us to think about beauty globally and about the ways it travels, producing certain forms of affect that transcend boundaries and which enable transnational biopolitical operations that are tied to both colonial histories and new forms of empire. I propose that the twin concepts of biopolitics and affect can be applied to many different contexts where beauty matters, and that they allow us to think beyond the structure/agency or empowerment/disempowerment debates that have long plagued academic discussions of beauty practices.

CHAPTER I

The Eugenesis of Beauty

At the beginning of the twentieth century, Brazil was undergoing a process of rapid industrialization and urbanization. The country was controlled by an alliance of landowner oligarchies and educated urban elites, which sought to modernize the country but did not want the process to threaten the rigid social hierarchies that had propelled these groups into positions of power. The phrase inscribed in the new Brazilian flag, "Order and Progress," typified the elites' desire for both economic progress and an intact social order. Although the period known as the Old Republic was inaugurated by both the official abolition of slavery in 1888 and the transition from a monarchy into a liberal republic in 1889, there were few real changes in the structure of power during that period. First, the new constitution of 1891 determined that only male literate citizens were eligible to vote and hold office, which excluded a large majority of the population from democratic participation.[1] Second, abolition did little to change the situation of the black population in Brazil, because the economic structure reserved only the lowest-paying jobs for them.

The historian Kim Butler has argued that state and private incentives for white immigration, resulting in the arrival of an average of fifteen thousand European immigrants a year from 1850 to 1930, pushed most Afro-Brazilians out of the best-remunerated positions in the agricultural and industrial economies, particularly in the southeast. Recognizing the inevitable end to the slave economy, many plantation owners stopped buying slaves and refused to employ freepersons, arguing that these workers were inherently indolent; they preferred immigrant workers instead.[2] This meant that even though Afro-Brazilians had formed the backbone of an exploitative colonial economy, they were systematically excluded from any real opportunities for upward mobility.

Along with the economic transformations taking place, there arose new imaginaries of the Brazilian nation that were profoundly shaped by a eugenic understanding of sanitation and improvement of the population. The educated members of the elite were avid readers and admirers of European scientific thought, but they did not necessarily share the negative social-Darwinist view of Brazil espoused by many European intellectuals. For instance, Count Joseph Arthur de Gobineau, a French emissary in Brazil and one of the first to promote the concept of Aryan superiority, wrote that Brazil was condemned to backwardness owing to widespread miscegenation. He declared that its people were "a completely mulatto population, polluted in the blood and the spirit, and frighteningly ugly."[3]

Afrânio Peixoto, an influential professor of public health and legal medicine, had a strong response for Gobineau in his book *Climate and Health: A Bio-Geographical Introduction to Brazilian Civilization*:

> In 1869, while in Brazil, Gobineau predicted that "children are dying in such high quantities that in the matter of a few, negligible years, there will be no more Brazilians." . . . Not only is the Brazilian population growing enormously . . . but racial mixture is also rapidly increasing. The white albumen is purifying the national molasses. . . . Pure blacks do not exist anymore; mestizos disappear, either because they die prematurely due to somatic weaknesses, sensuality, nervousness and sensitivity to tuberculosis, or because they interbreed with whiter elements: thus the race whitens. . . . In Brazil, the great race—that has assimilated and distilled the other two races, *which are only undesirable due to their uncultured condition and ugliness*— is the white race. . . . Every day morbidity and mortality surrender to the sanitation of housing and of urban settings, in such a way that currently our mortality rate has a very dignified standing among the best in the world.[4]

Peixoto counters Gobineau's pessimistic evaluation of Brazil by declaring that miscegenation is not the problem but rather the solution to Brazil's problems. Using a different eugenic logic than Gobineau, he argues that mortality rates had been lowered through sanitation, and that if any lower types remain, they will naturally disappear because they are unfit. Thus, with ongoing racial mixture only the white race prevails, whitening the nation as a whole. Both Gobineau and Peixoto, however, seem to agree on the fact that ugliness is a mark of being dysgenic and thus biopolitically undesirable—Peixoto is simply more optimistic that the ugly elements of the Brazilian population will be weeded out.

Peixoto was not alone in putting forward the whitening thesis—at the turn of the century, miscegenation began to be consistently portrayed by the Brazilian intelligentsia as a constructive force that would create a racially homogeneous country in the long run, particularly if it was combined with sanitation campaigns and the proper moral and hygienic education. The power of medicine was understood as capable of rooting ugliness out of the population, an ugliness that was a marker of disease, ignorance, and vice rather than simply an aesthetic evaluation of different physiognomies. The ongoing mixture between white men and indigenous and African women, on the other hand, promised to improve the nation's racial stock, which would be visible in the beauty of the children produced from such unions. Beauty became a sign of the nation's racial improvement, and ugliness became a sign of what needed to be corrected in Brazil.

Eugenic thought, in other words, produced the backbone of the aesthetic hierarchy present to this day in Brazil, which pronounces certain bodies more beautiful and therefore more valuable than others, and which cherishes the power of beautification practices to elevate individuals within that hierarchy. It was one of the leading eugenicists, Renato Kehl, who first promoted plastic surgery as a valuable tool that could complement the work of eugenics in the effort to improve the Brazilian population. The title of this chapter is a play on words: the word *eugenesis,* defined as the condition of being eugenic, draws attention to the ways in which beauty became a marker for eugenic improvement, but it is also reminiscent of the word *genesis,* suggesting that this historical moment inaugurated beauty's ongoing centrality to the national project.

VISUALIZING UGLINESS

The Brazilian intelligentsia of the postabolition period was not always confident about the nation's future. The small white elite that controlled the country felt threatened by a large majority that was uneducated, extremely poor, and of mixed race, and were unsure whether there were enough white immigrants coming in from Europe to offset the dark-skinned masses. For example, Raimundo Nina Rodrigues, a doctor and anthropologist who wrote extensively on the racial question in Brazil in the late nineteenth century, originally shared the pessimism of Europeans with regard to Brazil, believing racial mixture would inevitably lead to degeneration and increased crime, particularly in the poorer northeastern regions of the country.[5] One can perceive a subtle shift in his writings, however, toward the end of his career, when he began to give the environment a more important role than race in Brazil's future.[6]

His students at the Medical School of Bahia, such as Afrânio Peixoto, shed most of this racial pessimism in the following decades and instead sought to emphasize the plasticity of the Brazilian nation and its people. There was a marked change in popular-culture narratives as well. One of the key foundational fictions of Brazil, *Os Sertões* (Rebellion in the Backlands) by Euclides da Cunha (published in 1902), describes Brazil's northeastern rural population as sickly, indolent, and dangerous and simultaneously highlights the potential of this population to become civilized and productive members of the nation.[7] The writer Monteiro Lobato followed suit in 1918, inventing an archetypal figure known as Jeca Tatu, an ignorant and lethargic rural worker who, upon encountering hygienic education and sanitation measures, became an industrious, healthy, and exemplary worker.[8]

The shift away from racial pessimism was the product of a new form of eugenic thinking that rejected the notion that climate and race would destine the nation to indolence and poverty, and instead proclaimed that it was disease, ignorance, and vice that were at the root of Brazil's unproductivity. It was a form of scientific racism insofar as its explicit aim was to racially improve the nation, but it was an approach significantly different from that espoused by German or American eugenics, which sought to prevent racial mixing as well as the reproduction of the unfit. The historian Nancy Leys Stepan has described it as a neo-Lamarckian eugenics that "often came tinged with an optimistic expectation that reforms of the social milieu would result in permanent improvement, an idea in keeping with the environmentalist-sanitary tradition that had become fashionable."[9] This optimism was based on recent advancements in Brazilian microbiology, particularly the international recognition given to the Oswaldo Cruz Institute after its successful sanitation and vaccination campaigns in Rio de Janeiro against the bubonic plague, yellow fever, and smallpox. The director of the institute, Oswaldo Cruz, became a "cultural hero among the elite" because he seemed to prove not only that the country could produce scientific innovation but also that public health initiatives backed by the state could do away with many of the obstacles that seemed to hold the nation back in relation to others.[10] This new paradigm reflected a newfound faith in medical science and a vision of the Brazilian population as malleable and perfectible.

Notions of beauty and ugliness played a central role in neo-Lamarckian eugenics. Medical discourses on ugliness preceded discourses on beauty, because ugliness was a key way to demarcate biopolitical others who were seen as a threat to the nation. Carlos Chagas, who was then a student of Oswaldo Cruz, gained national notoriety after discovering the pathogenesis of a disease that became a symbol of the poor state of health of rural Brazilians, and which was theorized as a probable cause for their general unproductivity. This illness, which came to be known as Chagas's disease, was said to affect at least 2 million rural workers, at a time when the total population of Brazil had barely reached 30 million. More importantly for my argument, however, was how Chagas described the sufferers of the illness at the 1912 Medical Congress in Belo Horizonte: "As a rule, those infected with the most severe cases do not reach adulthood, disappearing early on for the collective benefit; when the illness allows them to reach an older age, however, it stunts their physical development, thus resulting in miserable creatures of monstrous appearance, who are an assault against the beauty of life and against the harmony of things in those [rural] regions."[11]

We see here the eugenic reassurance that the weakest will simply disappear for the collective benefit of the nation, but also the dire warning that if the state does not intervene with public health initiatives, there will only be more "creatures of monstrous appearance" populating the rural landscape. Chagas instrumentalized ugliness, in other words, as a way to garner sympathy for the populations he sought to treat, but also as a way to aestheticize the threat of those afflicted by disease, portraying them as an assault against the very senses of his urban audience. His ultimate goal was to expand, to the national level, the scope and influence of the Oswaldo Cruz Institute, which until then had acted mostly in southeastern urban settings, and this required a hyperbolic description of the rural areas as plagued by monstrous figures in desperate need of medical attention.

Other members of the Oswaldo Cruz Institute shared similar objectives. In 1912 the institute sponsored the nine-month scientific expedition of two doctors, Belisário Penna and Arthur Neiva, through the northeastern and central regions of Brazil in order to chronicle the state of poor rural workers. Like the reports yielded by other naturalists' expeditions before it, Penna and Neiva's report also catalogued the flora and the fauna of the *sertões*, or "backlands," but it was the body of the rural worker that became a central object of scrutiny and concern in the report and in later discussions about it. What most shocked the reading

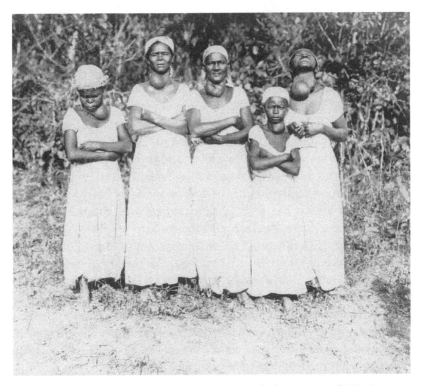

FIG 2. Women and girls afflicted with gout, photographed on Penna and Neiva's scientific expedition. Photo courtesy of Memórias do Instituto Oswaldo Cruz.

public at the time were the photographs that accompanied the report and which graphically depicted the dire state of the health of the population in rural areas. Consider the example in fig. 2.

The photographs taken by Penna and Neiva concentrated on visible signs of disease, such as goiter, and sought to visually connect physical abnormalities to the sorry state of the black rural population. Photography had been used in Brazil since the nineteenth century to visualize the black body as a laboring or deviant body, as Beatriz Rodriguez Balanta has cogently argued,[12] but Penna and Neiva also sought to explicitly connect this body to medical deformities. The captions for the photographs, on the other hand, comment frequently on the backwardness or lack of intelligence of the photographic subjects. A photograph of a woman with a slight case of goiter has the following caption: "The size of the goiter does not always correlate with intellectual depression: this photograph represents an ill woman bearing a multi-lobar goiter of small dimensions, yet demonstrating very poor intellect." The photograph of a man with a severe case of goiter has a similar caption: "A bearer of goiter with a very low intellectual index. He presents, however, regular muscular development."[13] The emphasis on intelligence seems to suggest that disease affects intellectual development to different degrees, but the caption offers hope that this correlation is not inevitable, and that goiter may not affect the rural workers' physical ability to till the land.

The report's long discussion of diseases that are less visible on the body, such as malaria and yellow fever, and their relative absence from the expedition's photographic record in comparison to goiter, indicate that these photographs of goiter perform several key functions. First, as Nancy Leys Stepan has pointed out, they provide visual evidence to back up Carlos Chagas's claim that the etiology of goiter is related to advanced Chagas's disease, a claim later proven to be false.[14] A visible deformity such as goiter served as an aesthetic marker of difference for these rural bodies, a deformity that was meant to cause a sense of aesthetic repulsion among Penna and Neiva's educated readers. This dichotomy between the observer and the observed reinforced the social differences between the ruling elites and the Brazilian working class: the educated observer was expected to examine, measure, and appraise the healthiness or unhealthiness of the subject in question.

Second, linking a visible deformity such as goiter to intellectual ability was a subtle way to racialize the subjects of these photographs as an inferior type of human, unable to help themselves and thus in desperate need of biopolitical intervention to become civilized. The portrait of dark-skinned rural workers as deformed, stupefied, and nearly disabled by disease was part of a larger campaign to convince the political elites of the need for a more interventionist Brazilian state, for which public health should be a primary concern not only in metropolitan areas but also in locales neglected until then.[15] The starkness of the report was said to have inspired Miguel Pereira, one of the founders of the sanitation movement, to declare in 1916: "Outside of Rio de Janeiro and São Paulo, now more or less sanitized cities[,] . . . Brazil is still a vast hospital. . . . Chagas's genius discovery has revealed to the country . . . a Dantesque spectacle of generations upon generations of malformed individuals and paralytics, of cretins and idiots."[16]

Belisário Penna would go on to publish a series of articles in the newspaper *Correio da Manhã* in his efforts to influence public opinion on the need for sanitation, articles that were then reprinted in his book *Saneamento do Brasil* (The Sanitation of Brazil). In those articles, he argues repeatedly that during his travels he witnessed widespread physical and intellectual infirmity among the rural population, painting a desolate picture in which nearly everyone is ill with one disease or another: "In certain localities no one, literally no one from the area escapes . . . infection. These are small towns of one hundred to three hundred inhabitants, where there is merely a vegetative, animalistic way of life, and where entire families are made up of crippled, retarded and goitered semi-idiotic individuals, this in areas with luxurious vegetation, fertile lands, crystalline waters and healthy climates."[17] Although Penna and Neiva were unable to conduct full diagnostic exams in the field, Penna asserts that the very visibility of sickness on the bodies of the rural populace, in sharp contrast to the idyllic environment where these people lived, was enough to confirm their diseased state.

For Penna, human ugliness became a blemish in what would otherwise be a beautiful and productive Brazilian landscape, marking rural workers as the very vectors of disease that the nation must target in order to heal itself. His discourse about these bodies made visible a frontier that was yet to be sanitized and medicalized—the diseased body of the backlands. Whereas Penna and Neiva's original report favored a more scientific and neutral language while cataloguing the diseases of the backlands, Penna's newspaper articles adopt a much more hyperbolic language that does not shy away from nearly apocalyptic imagery. These hyperbolic descriptions were clearly meant to rouse support in favor of a national sanitation movement, and Penna specifically calls for state intervention: "The primordial and utmost concern of conscious government leaders should be the physical, moral and intellectual sanitation of its inhabitants."[18] Penna presented sanitation as a matter of national interest to his readers, not only because sanitation would address the diseases that prevented national progress, but also because it would provide "real incorporation into civilization" for those "ignorant individuals" abandoned to their fate.[19]

Although Penna claims repeatedly that climate and race are not the reason for Brazil's problems, and he promises the full rehabilitation of poor rural workers through sanitation and hygiene, he also racializes their current state by blaming it on the end of slavery:

These thousands of ignorant and rude individuals, freed from the not always humane yoke [of slavery], dispersed in all directions, descended by the legions upon the forests and backlands, onto the margins of rivers and streams. They then gave in to alcohol and to orgies, without the least notion of hygiene, becoming animalized and nearly returning to the savage state of their forefathers in their natural desire to fully use their freedom—a freedom whose delights they were unable to comprehend and which can only be enjoyed through work, through methodical effort and by cultivating one's spirit and one's health. All these people, when they were still slaves, were subject to work discipline, were generally well fed, and were relatively well taken care of and sheltered, for this was in the primordial interest of plantation owners.[20]

The language of racial degeneration is clear in this quote—without the guidance of the educated Brazilians, former slaves return to their savage state and become animalized, giving in to vices and unbridled desire. Although Penna does not advocate a return to slavery, this passage makes clear both his idealization of slavery as a paternalistic form of care for slaves, and his nostalgia for a simpler time when plantation owners were able to assert their public authority over the working population. In the absence of this authority, which had suddenly ceased after the abolition of slavery in 1888, Penna calls for the Brazilian State to step in and, in the name of hygiene, reorganize the rural working class into a productive force. Leaving this population to their own devices would only cause their own degeneration and, consequently, would arrest the progress of the nation as a whole.

Penna's urgent message was based on his apprehension regarding the economic changes Brazil was undergoing. As the historian Gilberto Hochman points out, Belisário Penna was a traditionalist who criticized the artificiality of fostering urban industries when the natural Brazilian economic activity, in his eyes, would always be agriculture.[21] For Penna, one of the worst consequences of the rapid expansion of urban industry was the wave of migration it was stimulating from rural to metropolitan areas. As the impoverished peripheries of Brazilian cities began to grow, other sanitarists, like Afrânio Peixoto, would argue that the backlands and their endemic rural diseases were now much closer to the general population, and that the need to sanitize the country was even more urgent than before.

The sanitation movement, Hochman argues, thus redefined the borders between rural and metropolitan areas: "For the pro-sanitation campaign, the *sertões* [backlands] and rural areas were more of a medical, social and political category than a geographic location. Their spatial location would depend on the existence of the pairing of disease and neglect. Therefore, the *sertões* would not be as far removed from those who would decide on sanitation measures, nor would they merely be a symbolic or geographic reference to the country's interior."[22] The *sertões* were located wherever the rural working-class body was located. As the country became transformed by mass urbanization, the sick body that was first imagined as an isolated rural predicament came to be understood as a vector of disease that was expanding and becoming a threat to all Brazilians. Wherever rural migrants settled in their search for jobs, they would bring their illnesses and meager hygiene, which would be neatly visible on their bodies as a form of ugliness, according to the sanitarists.

REPRODUCING BEAUTY

If ugliness racialized rural workers as inferior and sickly, beauty served as its mirror image and became a highly desirable trait that marked the superiority of the Brazilian elites. The ability to produce and reproduce beauty within urban populations, therefore, became a central concern for the Brazilian intelligentsia—how could they be assured that their favorable traits would be passed on to the following generations? The answer was once again eugenics, particularly Francis Galton's brand of eugenics, which was popularized in Brazil through the writings of Dr. Renato Kehl. Despite being significantly younger than Afrânio Peixoto and Belisário Penna, Renato Kehl gained their admiration after he founded the Eugenic Society of São Paulo in 1918 and began to correspond with them about how to promote this new science among other educated Brazilians.[23] Eventually, Kehl created a network of eugenics advocates that extended throughout Brazil and even beyond its borders, demonstrated by his ability to organize the First Brazilian Eugenics Congress in 1929, which included delegates from Argentina, Peru, Chile, and Paraguay. That same year, he founded the Central Brazilian Commission of Eugenics and began to publish a monthly journal, the *Bulletin of Eugenics,* both of which sought to educate Brazilians regarding eugenic ideology and influence Brazilian legislation regarding marriage and immigration.[24] Kehl, in other words, is a key figure who influenced the shape and form that eugenics took in Brazil.

Almost all of Renato Kehl's writings focus on beauty and identify it as both the aim of eugenic practice and the product of proper hygiene and sanitation. Take, for instance, his definition of eugenics at the beginning of his first book, *Eugenics and Social Medicine,* published in 1920: "What is eugenics? Eugenics is the science of good reproduction. It does not attempt, as many believe, to simply avoid the agglomeration of ugly people. Its objectives are not restricted to Kalipedia, that is, to having beautiful children. Beauty is a eugenic ideal. Galton's science, however, does not have limited horizons. . . . Eugenics is not restricted to elevating exterior perfection. It makes visible this exterior, but its acute vision desires the complete representation of perfection, culminating in somatic and moral beauty."[25] In this passage, Kehl explains that eugenics produces beautiful forms among the next generations, but that this beauty is a sign of something more profound—an interior as well as an exterior perfection, a symbol of an individual's health and moral rectitude.

Kehl goes on to explain that hygienic and eugenic practices will positively select the best attributes of the human race, improving and beautifying humanity as a whole. Those practices include educating the public about how to intelligently choose a spouse and introducing laws that prohibit unfit marriages among the less educated.[26] To justify these policies, he reminds his readers of the dire state of affairs of the Brazilian rural population, the "pariahs who aside from being illiterate are also mentally retarded, true cretins, as was observed by Belisário Penna and Arthur Neiva."[27] For Kehl, the more restrictive reproductive policies would be clearly limited to these pariahs, the inferior elements of the Brazilian population; he believed the Brazilian elites were more than able to apply on their own the right criteria while choosing a spouse.

The reproduction of beauty through eugenic means was a highly gendered ideology. Kehl felt that eugenic practices would look different for men and for women, and that these practices would have different effects as well. In the case of men, Kehl was mostly worried about the fitness of men in the Brazilian military. In a section titled "Eugenics and Militarism" in *Eugenics and Social Medicine,* Kehl laments that dysgenic qualities have sapped the strength of young men: "The average value of Brazilian youth is of inferior quality. I do not deny youth its patriotism, bravery and intrepidness—these qualities are not lacking. What is scarce among it is strong and healthy representatives. . . . Repair how the national type is in general ugly and frail—we are of good fiber, bringing the vital patrimony of our grandfathers, but illnesses threaten to derail us. The ugly, the deviant, the degenerate are abundant in great proportions in our country, and attempt to influence maliciously the future of our nationality."[28]

The historian Maria Bernardete Ramos Flores has argued that the sense of inferiority that the Brazilian intelligentsia felt in relation to other countries was frequently expressed as a "crisis of virility," whereby the backwardness caused by vice, sickness, and disorder was seen as a negative feminization of the population.[29] I would add that this crisis of virility was also equated with ugliness, because Kehl believed degeneration would show on the physiques of the men in question—associating frailty with nonwhite bodies. In a short study titled *A Healthy People and an Ailing People,* Kehl adopted an anthropometric approach to determine an "index of robustness," calculated by subtracting one's weight and thoracic width from one's height, and in this way determined mathematically that young Brazilian men enlisting for the army were physically inferior to those enlisting in other countries.[30] He also offered hope, however, demonstrating that after medical treatment with vermicide there was a lower incidence of anemia and "a significant difference between the muscular strength of sick individuals and the strength of the same individuals days after being cured."[31] Illness was not destiny but an obstacle to be defeated, and thus the Brazilian population could be remasculinized.

Kehl did not, however, focus on the details of male bodies in the same way that he focused on female bodies: their ideal measurements, the many reasons for their inadequacies, and the eugenic techniques available to improve them. While, for Kehl, male beauty seems to mainly imply health, strength, and fitness, female beauty is a more intractable issue that requires many more interventions on the body. In one of his longest and most important books, *The Cure of Ugliness,* Kehl spends much more time addressing how one produces "feminine plastic perfection" than discussing male beauty. He clearly imagines most of his readers as educated males, who would have a strong interest in fostering the beauty of their daughters or female protégés: "Ugliness can be avoided and cured. It is up to parents and to educators, in great measure, to avoid it. Many ugly maidens, lacking in grace, owe their misfortune to morbid perversions, or to personal carelessness."[32]

The central argument of this book is that ugliness is not simply an expression of immutable inherited characteristics but a disharmony caused by illness, vice, or psychic abnormalities, and therefore ugliness can and should be removed from the body. Kehl's focus on female beauty, particular the beauty of unmarried young women, signals how central they were for the national eugenic project—they would engender the next generation of Brazilians and would be in charge of these children's care and early education. Kehl's message about beauty was a double-edged sword, however, since it implied that wealthy Brazilian families, already anxious about marrying off their daughters, were to blame for their daughters' aesthetic failings. What if, despite adopting all the prophylactic measures that Kehl recommended in *The Cure of Ugliness,* such as healthy eating habits, wholesome psychological development, good personal hygiene, dedication to physical education and general care for the body, the women of these families still exhibited unpleasing aesthetic characteristics?

Perhaps preempting this objection, Renato Kehl embraced a medical technology that was still controversial at the time in Brazil: plastic surgery. The first beauty clinics were opened in Rio de Janeiro and São Paulo in the 1920s, but very few, if any, offered cosmetic treatments that required surgical intervention. Mainstream medical practice did not yet accept plastic surgery as a valid medical technique. Kehl, however, regarded plastic surgery as a very promising medical discipline that would perfectly complement his neo-Lamarckian eugenic science, since both regarded the body as malleable and perfectible.[33]

In *The Cure of Ugliness,* Kehl dedicates a whole chapter to the benefits of plastic surgery, and he discusses in great detail how surgery could remove wrinkles, correct sagging or enlarged breasts, and create more beautiful features. For example, this is how he evaluates nose jobs, or rhinoplasties: "The progress in the domain of rhinoplasty is really admirable. And thanks to it, how many deformities will our sight be spared? How many young girls that are robust and have perfect bodies, but who have deformed noses, would refuse to get their noses reformed in Greek or Roman style, for their own delight and the delight of their admirers?"[34] This passage is revealing because it emphasizes solely female beauty. Despite the fact that men, too, could benefit from rhinoplasties, plastic surgery is portrayed as more appropriate for women, who are objects of admiration for the male gaze. Kehl portrays the upper-class female body as one that would require medical interventions throughout its entire life to correct even small flaws and to constantly fight the effects of aging. Kehl reassures his readers that despite the relative novelty of plastic surgery within the Brazilian context, it was already widely accepted in European countries such as Germany, with excellent results. It is unclear from his writings whether Kehl believed that the benefits of plastic surgery were inheritable, but he unequivocally endorsed it as a eugenic practice that could treat "perfectly removable deformities."[35]

Kehl's work extended the biopolitical use of beauty and ugliness that Belisário Penna and the sanitarists had begun, since it went beyond diagnosing the dysgenic qualities of rural populations and began to equate beautification with Brazil's eugenic progress in all spheres of life and among all populations. Compared to the sanitarists, Kehl had less faith that the Brazilian masses could be redeemed simply through medical intervention, declaring that "due to its state of morbidity, the national citizenry is generally ugly, squalid, weak and diminished, and unable to compete with foreigners."[36] Kehl's mention of foreigners is key here, since he strongly supported additional immigration from Europe in order to whiten the national population.

Kehl believed miscegenation would lead to the gradual disappearance of nonwhite races:

> In Brazil, we observed an intense mixture between the three races that inhabit it, and if we accept Novicow's idea that the superior ones will subjugate the inferior ones, with the consequent increase in offspring of the superior types and gradual disappearance of the inferior races, we will verify in time the extinction of the black and the rainforest-dwelling races. . . . We can affirm that Brazil is advancing toward perfecting its population, until it is constituted by a strong, vigorous and intellectually superior race. . . . The mulatto [the offspring of a European and an African], the *mameluco* [the offspring of a European and an Amerindian] and the *cafuso* [the offspring of an African and Amerindian] are in general ugly human types. There have been known to be some beautiful mulattas and mulattos, but they are the exception rather than the rule.[37]

Beautification, for Kehl, was unequivocally associated with whitening. He disparaged the indigenous and black populations of Brazil as inferior races destined to disappear, and considered mixed-race populations to be generally ugly. Only mulattas and mulattos could, on rare occasions, be beautiful specimens, according to Kehl, and thus perfectible and worthy of a reproductive future. He was crafting an aesthetic hierarchy where whiteness was clearly the most desirable and dominant quality, and where racialization went hand-in-hand with aesthetic evaluations of the body.

THE EROTICS OF MISCEGENATION

By the 1930s, eugenic ideals had become widespread among Brazil's reading public and had influenced legislation, public health measures, medical research, novels, and even educational manuals. Kehl, for example, wrote a children's book, *Hygeia the Fairy: Your First Book on Hygiene*, which introduced elementary school children to basic hygienic practices and was officially adopted as required reading by the Board of Directors of Public Instruction of several Brazilian states. Borrowing from eugenic discourse, in fact, was a way to legitimize a wide variety of new publications and new fields of study, no matter how risqué.

Brazilian sexology was at the time a nascent branch of medicine, one not fully accepted by mainstream medicine but very popular among lay readers owing to the suggestive topics covered, which had previously been taboo. Publishers perceived the sales potential of these new writers and regularly added photographic and painted female nudes to the books in an effort to attract new readers.[38] The most famous and most widely read sexologist was Hernani de Irajá, who was born in 1897 in the southern state of Rio Grande do Sul but who practiced medicine most of his life in Rio de Janeiro. A prolific writer, he wrote more than thirty books about sexuality between the 1920s and the 1960s, most of which were reprinted several times and went through several editions. The central argument of his work is that sexuality should be a subject of serious scientific analysis, because it can become a fundamental tool in bringing about the "moral and physical eugenesis of the race."[39] Although Irajá never achieved the recognition that was awarded to Kehl or the sanitarists, his work is significant because it provides insight into the ways that scientific and erotic discourses about race became intermingled in the Brazilian imagination.

The aim of Irajá's sexological writings is twofold: they map out the differences between normal and abnormal sexual behavior and provide a typology of Brazilian women, ranking them from the least to the most desirable. His imagined readership clearly was educated Brazilian males, for whom choosing the appropriate sexual partners should be a matter of concern, since it would determine the future of not only their family but also the nation as a whole. In *Morphology of Woman: Female Plasticity in Brazil,* Irajá explains to his readers that unlike other nations, such as China or Russia, Brazil is a complicated fusion of different nations, a "people still in formation and subject to modification."[40] Central to Irajá's argument is his belief that sexual selection could unlock Brazil's untapped potential or condemn its fate.

Irajá ranks women who live in rural areas as less desirable than urban women. Following the same neo-Lamarckian arguments given by the sanitarists, he argues that disease, poverty, and physical work had left legible marks on the bodies of these women:

> There is a lack of artistic harmony in the populations that are poorly fed and overburdened by everyday labor. . . . Their characteristics betray their general discomfort. Their features, generally graceful in younger women, intermix with premature wrinkles that appear on the skin due to their everyday urgencies and difficulties. . . . Their collarbones protrude in excess, their emaciated hands resemble the simian type, their bony feet denote the vestiges of hyperhidrosis or have been deformed by martyrizing shoes. In rural areas the common *bicho do pé* [chigoe flea] adds to these ills, producing veritable monstrosities.[41]

The desolate portrait of these women is meant to produce not only empathy but also an aesthetic revulsion in the reader. The health and happiness of these women had been compromised by their working and health conditions, but their beauty seemed to have suffered most of all, transforming what could have been graceful women into "veritable monstrosities." The term *simian* also racializes them, but it links that racialization to their condition rather than to steadfast hereditary causes. To make the contrast clearer, Irajá points out that "the affluent classes, exempt from these or other circumstances—misery, nutritional deficiencies, etc.—are the ones which possess the best morphologically wrought specimens."[42]

Irajá goes on to generate a Brazilian geography of beauty, trying to determine which regions of the country have the most beautiful types. Based on the statistics produced by the Brazilian military service, he argues that human specimens in the southern region of Brazil present more robust characteristics, owing to the presence of purer white types and less mixture with inferior elements. In contrast, the northern and central regions of Brazil are less eugenic, owing to more widespread miscegenation with indigenous and African elements. Irajá also claims to have conducted his own anthropometric studies of women from different regions of Brazil, in which he measured the proportion of the dimensions of the head to the individual's overall height, following aesthetic canons first developed by Greek sculptors and then developed by Renaissance artists.

The emphasis on scientific measurements allows Irajá to naturalize these differences as objective medical truths, not subjective judgments. He writes,

> The svelte or long type is the most aristocratic. In general, the height exceeds 1m62 [five feet four inches]. Brazil possesses marvelous examples of this class, widespread among Indo-European mixtures. The cities . . . of southern Brazil are rich in beauties of this "elancé" type that stands 7 1/2 heads high. The short or squat type is more bourgeois. It belongs to the working classes of the fields or the factories. However, when there is a perfect equilibrium in the plastic disposition of the trunk, head and members, the short type is particularly charming and graceful, light and agile. . . . In Ceará, Pernambuco and other northeastern states, one can find true "beauties" in the mixture of that originally indigenous type with the Dutch, the Portuguese or even the English.[43]

These typologies created by Irajá serve the purpose of educating the male reading public about the most eugenically appropriate spouses, at the same time that they reinforce the regional, racial, and class hierarchies in

Brazil. The southern urban population is described as having abundant beautiful women owing to its European background, while the mixed-race women of lower classes, rural areas, and the northeastern states are described as shorter, but charming or beautiful on rare occasions, particularly when they have clear European heritage.

Irajá's text is accompanied by dozens of female nudes, either photographs of nudes taken in a studio or nudes Irajá drew himself, as well as a few photographs of seminude indigenous men and women surrounded by vegetation. The photographs of indigenous peoples come with little explanation other than the names the groups they belong to, performing a type of ethnographic journey through the Brazilian landscape and resembling a museum-like experience of portraying racial Otherness.[44] The other female nudes, however, are nearly pornographic in their eroticism and portray young women in sensual poses, invitingly looking at the camera or stretched out on a bed. These women are described in detail in the captions, focusing on their height, the quality of their hair, the firmness of their breasts, any diseases they might suffer from, and invariably, their racial type. All these women are described as European or as racially mixed (using the word *morena* [brown] or *mestiça* [mestizo]), but most of them are light-skinned.

The example in fig. 3 is interesting because it shows a clear discursive contrast side-by-side on the same page. The figure on the left is described as a "mixed national type" with "predominant 'afer' characteristics, despite the cutaneous depigmentation." Despite her light skin, in other words, she can be recognized as primarily Homo sapiens afer, a racist term Irajá borrows from Linnaeus to describe people of African descent.[45] Irajá clearly considers her a dysgenic type because she has "small, atrophied breasts" and suffers from ovarian dysfunction. The figure on the right, in contrast, is described as a "French type" with "small, flattened breasts of good plasticity," and no signs of disease.[46] Irajá is educating the reader, in other words, to view secondary racial characteristics, besides skin color, as markers of underlying eugenic or dysgenic qualities. Both of these women are presented as objects of sexual desire, but one would produce a better lineage than the other.

Irajá's preference for whiteness, however, does not contradict his message that female beauty should be cherished even if it is racially mixed, particularly because in that case it is something exceptional and uncommon. The reader, the one who consumes these erotic photographs and drawings, is imagined as a white Brazilian male belonging to the elite, who can redeem these lower types through reproduction.

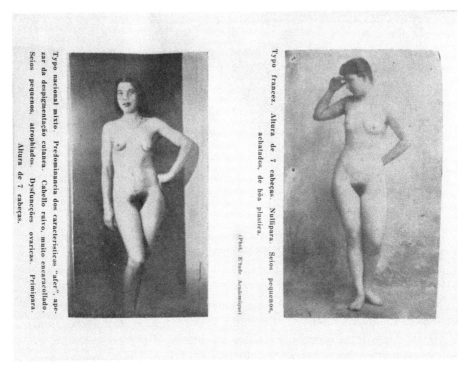

FIG 3. A comparison of body types in Irajá's *Morphology of Woman.*

Irajá's concluding chapter in *Morphology of Woman* explicitly conveys this message in a graph presented as an equation (see fig. 4). This equation translates as "Black Woman + Indigenous Woman + White Man = Light-Skinned Woman." Given Irajá's aesthetic hierarchy, we can safely assume he believed this light-skinned woman to be eugenically superior and more beautiful than the woman who bore her. The narrative here is one in which white men have the power to whiten and thus eugenically improve the nation, by producing offspring with less privileged women of other races. As Irajá put it: "The Aryanization of the Brazilian is an inevitable law confirmed by logic."[47] Furthermore, Irajá naturalizes white male desire for mixed-race women in the book *Sex and Beauty* by arguing that scientific measurements have determined that mulattas have bigger buttocks, and "a woman with developed hips and great buttocks is considered in most populations as more apt for fecundation, gestation and giving birth. . . . [I]nstinct almost always aids sexual selection."[48] The desire to eugenically improve the nation through

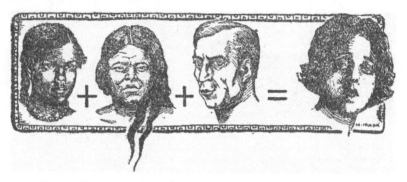

FIG 4. An equation presented in Irajá's *Morphology of Woman.*

reproduction is equated here with sexual instinct—thus naturalizing the white male desire for nonwhite beauty.

Irajá's narrative is silent about the taboo possibility that a white woman from the elite might conceive children with a dark-skinned man, but we can assume he would consider such a combination not only morally unacceptable but also a step toward degeneration rather than whitening. Irajá warns his readers repeatedly of psychological deviations that prompt women to be anything but dedicated housewives and mothers. He preferred women to be delicate and passive and was particularly concerned with masculinized women who practiced too many sports, since he believed it might lead to homosexual propensities.

Young women from good families, above all, had to be feminine and learn how to care for their beauty, consulting a doctor if they had any concerns about their weight or appearance:

> These young women should look for a specialist in nutritional diseases, or even better, a sexologist, so they are properly counseled to remedy the maladies that afflict them. Little defects of the face or hands . . . can bring great harm to girls who are slaves to aesthetic prejudice. They fixate on ideas. They imagine themselves to be observed and analyzed meticulously, just because they have a scar on their face, some hairs on their chin, a small mustache . . . an ear that protrudes a little, short fingers, fat hands. . . . Meanwhile, it never occurs to them or to their parents that an adequate treatment, sometimes a small, corrective aesthetic surgery that takes ten minutes, or a little psychoanalysis, can free them forever from obsessive thoughts or from uncomfortable anomalies.[49]

Even though Irajá argues that these women's aesthetic concerns are obsessive and unhealthy, his extensive list of defects has the precise effect of magnifying any anomalies under a meticulous medical gaze.

Ultimately, he advises, women and concerned parents should always defer to the expertise of medical authority to decide if aesthetic surgery or psychoanalysis is necessary. From his later writings, such as his legal defense of a surgery to reconstitute physical virginity by repairing broken hymens,[50] it becomes clear that he recommended aesthetic surgeries to his patients and perhaps carried them out himself. As a medical discipline, plastic surgery was rapidly becoming a marker of class privilege and a common recourse for well-to-do Brazilian women who wanted to hone their beauty and their femininity.

FREYRE'S NEO-LAMARCKISM

Brazilian historiography usually regards the scientific racism of the early twentieth century as having been checked by the publication, in 1933, of Gilberto Freyre's *Casa Grande e Senzala* (The Masters and the Slaves), a book of enormous impact in the Brazilian history of ideas. Trained in Columbia University under Franz Boas (who spearheaded the effort to delegitimize social Darwinism in the United States), Gilberto Freyre argued that the Aryanization of Brazil was not only untenable but also undesirable, because Brazil's hybrid culture, arising from the unique combination of African, Amerindian, and European elements, was the nation's most valuable asset. He privileged the erotic intimacy of colonial interactions within the private space of the plantation house, believing they enabled the fusion of distinct cultural practices and fostered a new Luso-tropical civilization that thrived and prospered within the Brazilian context.

Freyre certainly saw more potential in African and Amerindian populations than the eugenicists who preceded him, and he introduced the concept of cultural plasticity to delegitimize static conceptions of race. I think it is misguided, however, to consider his work to be a clean break from the past. First of all, following Ricardo Benzaquen de Araújo and Anadelia Romo, I regard his understanding of inheritance as explicitly neo-Lamarckian, like that of the sanitarists who came before him.[51] He explicitly argued that "the transmission of acquired characteristics" meant environmental adaptations could be inherited by future generations.[52] Second, the eugenicists had already touted miscegenation as a key aspect of Brazilian exceptionalism, and Freyre augmented that claim by adding culture to the mix. Third, Freyre's narrative consistently portrayed the nation as arising from the sexual union of European men with nonwhite women, mirroring the gendered and erotic aspects of miscegenation that were valued by eugenicists like Irajá. And finally, Freyre still valued beauty as a sign of the nation's ongoing improvement, like all the authors I have analyzed to this point.

Analyzing the continuities between Freyre and previous Brazilian thinkers, in other words, provides a more realistic portrait of both his influences and the Brazilian audience he was addressing. The biographer Pallares-Burke, for example, has remarked on Freyre's embrace of eugenic thought when he first wrote about Brazilian race relations in his 1922 master's thesis, stating his belief that the progress of the nation depended on a process of racial whitening.[53] Freyre was a product of his time, and even though he eventually tempered his message and abandoned the whitening thesis of the eugenicists in *Casa Grande e Senzala*, in my view he replaced it with a celebration of a Brazilian identity that was mostly European but which benefited from the "shadow, or at least the birthmark, of the aborigine or the negro."[54]

For example, Freyre talks of a new man of the tropics who was energized by black and indigenous blood, even as he was plagued by disease:

> The advantage of miscegenation coincided in Brazil with the enormous disadvantage of syphilis. They began together, one formed the Brazilian man—perhaps the ideal modern man for the tropics, a European energized by black or Indian blood—and the other one deformed him. Thus the confusion regarding responsibility, where many attributed to miscegenation what had been mainly caused by syphilis, blaming the Amerindians, the black race or even the Portuguese for the "ugliness" or "incapacity" of our mestizo populations most affected by syphilis or most gnawed by disease . . . when each of [these three races] are tired of producing admirable examples of beauty and robustness.[55]

In this passage, Freyre laments syphilis as a degenerative force in the Brazilian population that negated the positive effects of racial miscegenation. Freyre's persistent neo-Lamarckism allies him with the sanitarists, who had also argued that Brazil's problem was not a racial one but one of inadequate hygiene and meager public health. Like them, he argues that sanitizing the country would mean beautifying it, because there was nothing inherently dysgenic or unbeautiful about the racial components that made up Brazil's mestizo population. Inheritance and bodily aesthetics would be transformed by changing the environment.

Despite valuing the Amerindian and African elements of Brazilian identity, Freyre did not consider all racial groups as equal contributors to the national stock. For example, he paints a picture of indigenous populations as having been beautiful, healthy, and robust when the

Europeans first arrived on Brazilian shores, but sad, indolent, and weak after being enslaved to work in the sugarcane fields, losing the will to live as they became estranged from their original way of life.[56] They contributed to Brazilian customs and to the nation's culinary culture, but as their society deteriorated they had to be replaced with the more vigorous and more culturally advanced Africans. Freyre seems to naturalize the role of Africans within the colonial economy by arguing that they had a "biological and psychological predisposition for life in the tropics," remaining energetic and happy even under the harsh heat of the tropical sun.[57]

Not all African populations, however, were equal contributors to the nation. Freyre cites the contrast made by the eugenicist Oliviera Vianna between the "delicate features and relative beauty" of blacks in the state of Minas Gerais and the "simian appearance" of blacks in Rio de Janeiro in order to argue that Minas Gerais must have "imported a better black stock" to work in the mines.[58] Furthermore, Freyre equates beauty to cultural and individual development, making the case that the superior blacks in Minas Gerais must have originated in an African culture already familiar with metalwork, and that agricultural work simply required brute force, to which the inferior Hottentot Bushmen, with their "wide, flattened noses and enormous buttocks," were probably better suited.[59] Similarly, he argues that house slaves such as pages, maids, and cooks were "eugenically and aesthetically selected" for their greater height and attractiveness, and that because these female slaves had relations with white males they became mothers to "mulatto boys raised within the house, many of them future doctors, graduates and even priests."[60] Like Kehl, Freyre equates a better aesthetic appearance with more individual potential and with a better future for the nation.

In comparison to the African and Amerindian contributions to Brazilian society, which were mostly limited to culinary skill, personal hygiene, and physicality, the Portuguese are lauded in Freyre's work as a highly adaptable and plastic people who were, therefore, uniquely prepared for colonizing other lands. He claims the Portuguese were less religiously orthodox than the Spanish and less prejudiced than the English[61]—the other two colonizing forces of the Americas—and thus more willing to hybridize. He critiques those few Portuguese families in Brazil who sought to remain racially pure, because he claims it led to inbreeding and then to degenerative practices such as alcoholism.[62] Sensuality, according to Freyre, was the key to the colonizing process, a hypersensuality he attributes to the tropical climate in Brazil.[63] The Amerindian and African women became the conduits through which the Portuguese colonists learned how to live and love in the tropics and, thus, eventually evolve into Luso-tropical Brazilians.

Freyre does not portray the sexual violence of these unions, and instead sanitizes them by portraying these women as more than willing sexual partners, inescapably attracted to European men: "The milieu in which Brazilian life began was one of sexual intoxication. No sooner had the European leaped ashore than he found his feet slipping among the naked Indian woman. . . . The women were the first to offer themselves to the whites, the more ardent ones going to rub themselves against the legs of those beings whom they supposed to be gods. They would give themselves to the European for a comb or a broken mirror."[64] He similarly describes young mulattas as "initiating us [the sons of slave owners] in the ways of physical love . . . and providing us the first complete sensation of being a man."[65] Despite being critical of the cruelty of white Portuguese colonists toward African and Indian slaves in other passages, the narrative is clearly nostalgic for this mythical, almost Edenic time—the sexual intimacy that brings together the three races vindicates the violence of slavery. Freyre asserts, "It is unfair to accuse the Portuguese of having stained their grand work of tropical colonization with an institution that today we find repugnant. The place and the circumstances demanded slavery."[66] He then goes on to claim that the rigors of slavery were perhaps necessary to discipline the unruly energy of the African.

Freyre's origin story served the needs of nationalistic governments in both Brazil and Portugal. The Salazar government in Portugal embraced this version of history in order to argue that the Portuguese empire had established a more benign form of colonialism, since it allowed for racial and cultural hybridity.[67] The Vargas regime in Brazil, on the other hand, adopted traditionally Afro-Brazilian cultural expressions, like samba and Carnival, as national emblems that would now be the cultural property of all Brazilians.[68] By arguing that all ethnicities had come together in Brazil to forge a new common identity, Freyre pointed not only to a mythical past but also to a harmonious national future. This future would be marked by a common brownness, or *morenidade,* which Freyre describes as "a denial of race and an affirmation of metarace."[69]

In one of his few publications in English, *The Racial Factor in Contemporary Politics,* Freyre argues that Brazil's racial progressiveness is indexed by its tendency toward eugenic beauty: "Human aesthetic tastes in regard to human form and particularly to feminine beauty are being greatly affected by the increasing racial mixture that is going on, not only in large continental areas like Brazil, but in other areas as well. These are producing combinations of form and color that are no longer regarded with emphasis on their cacogenic, negative, effects, but on their sometimes impressively eugenic, and hence physically positive, aesthetic, effects. I belong to the number of those who think that this aesthetic aspect should not be underestimated."[70] Like other neo-Lamarckians before him, Freyre considered bodily aesthetics to be the measure of the eugenic advancement that Brazil had undergone—he simply believed the country was further along in the process than other eugenicists did. As late as 1984, Freyre defended the thesis that miscegenation between masters and their female slaves enacted the "anthropologically eugenic and aesthetic experiments" that regulated the saliencies of buttocks, thus "avoiding Africanoid exaggerations" in subsequent generations of Brazilians.[71] Miscegenation, in other words, has a teleological outcome—it produces eugenic beauty, regulating racial excess while simultaneously producing a more homogeneous body politic.

Of all the authors I analyze in this chapter, Gilberto Freyre is perhaps the only one who is still widely read in Brazil. *Casa Grande e Senzala* has been reedited more than fifty times, and Gilberto Freyre is widely considered one of the most important and influential social scientists in the history of Brazil. Despite the large number of critiques of his work—his sloppy historical methodology, his sanitization of slavery, his evacuation of economic relations to privilege personal relations,[72] to name only a few—many academics still staunchly defend his legacy. Hermano Vianna and David Lehman, for example, seek to reevaluate Freyre, and they critique the tendency to reduce Freyre to having created the myth of racial democracy when he never actually used the term in *Casa Grande e Senzala*.[73]

My purpose here is not to trace the larger impact of Freyre in the Brazilian history of ideas, or to describe how he is deployed in the current political context. Instead, I make the point that his celebration of racial mixture does not necessarily presume a complete rejection of eugenic ideals, because he reasserts the association between beauty and improvement of the national stock. As Barbara Weinstein and Jerry Dávila have both argued, the celebration of the Mãe Preta (Black Mother) in monuments and school textbooks, as a symbol of racial mixture and of black contributions to national identity, did not challenge the assumption that Brazil was a country leaving its black past behind and moving toward whiteness.[74] Both blackness and indigenousness are reduced to mere romanticized elements of Brazil's origin and do not determine its future. Whatever Freyre's intentions were with his writings, his celebration of hybridity and domestic racial intimacy were easily coopted by political discourses that pretended to promote racial equity in the national imaginary while reiterating older racial hierarchies. Thomas Skidmore suggests that this might explain why Freyre was so well received by the Brazilian intelligentsia and his book became an immediate sensation.[75]

EUGENIC LEGACIES

The objective of racially improving the nation through eugenic measures was not only a national project but also an individual one. Eugenics, as Kehl defined it, required that a man "make a balance of his life and verify whether there is an overall surplus or deficit, whether he is in organic condition to take on or restrain from marriage." He went on to state that "not everyone possesses the judgment necessary to make this evaluation. Thus, this task should be left to doctors."[76] The medical class took this task very seriously—they believed that the ultimate arbitration of what was beautiful, and therefore eugenic, should be left to them. Legally, however, very few restrictions were put on marriage licenses in Brazil, and sterilization was never approved as a government policy. It would seem eugenics had limited biopolitical applications in Brazil, compared to the United States and Europe.

Medical discourses about beauty, however, remained one of the main legacies of eugenic thinking in Brazil. Rather than limit reproduction, the neo-Lamarckian eugenics espoused by the Brazilian elites sought to map ugliness onto dysgenic properties of the body, and beauty onto eugenic qualities and virtues. Beauty was equated with hygiene, health, intelligence, and approximations to whiteness, and miscegenation began to be understood as a positive force that was irreversibly directing the nation toward a more eugenic future. The Brazilian intelligentsia had a duty to improve the health of the nation's citizens and to educate individuals on how to choose beautiful, eugenic spouses, but otherwise the nation was already on a path to a better future. Freyre reaffirmed this narrative about Brazil, reinterpreting the origin of the nation as the hybridization of the best eugenic qualities of the three races, which came together to create a new, more beautiful, Luso-tropical population. In short, the widespread notion that bodily aesthetics were a reliable index of the nation's improvement transformed beauty into a valuable biopolitical tool, one that could be applied to any individual or population to determine its worth.

Plastic surgery was the medical discipline that perhaps had most to gain from this conception of eugenic beauty, and the one that would carry forward this legacy in the decades to come. In 1933, the doctor who is now considered the "father" of plastic surgery in Brazil, José Rebello Neto, published a piece in the *Brazilian Journal of Otorhinolaryngology* defending this new discipline as a valid medical practice whose medical risks were worth taking. One of his main arguments was that plastic surgery is a eugenic practice, one that not only improves the individual psychological state of patients but also, by correcting small deformities, promotes the sexual union of undeniably eugenic young men and women and thus increases desirable maternity rates. He is clearly imagining plastic surgery as a tool for wealthier families, who would consider themselves already eugenic, yet still perfectible and in need of small corrections, particularly for their children of marriageable age. He also quotes Kehl's defense of plastic surgery in *The Cure of Ugliness* and finishes his article by stating: "It is certainly legitimate to accompany and encourage the march of humanity in search of an ideal of hygiene, eugenics and beauty! Plastic surgery is responsible for this lofty goal, which thus guarantees the brilliant place it occupies within the range of medical specialties."[77]

Plastic surgeons, therefore, began to imagine themselves as aiding not only their patients but also the nation as a whole, by bringing the entire population closer to eugenic ideals. The plastic surgery that Kehl embraced in 1923 took root in the country less than decade later, claiming its place as a key eugenic practice for the nation. Rebello Neto went on to open the first plastic surgery school in Brazil, as part of the Medical School of São Paulo, and founded the Brazilian Society of Plastic Surgery in 1948.[78] It was only in the 1960s, however, that plastic surgery began to be conceived as a right not only of the wealthy but also of the poor, expanding the target population that plastic surgeons wanted to beautify and improve upon.

CHAPTER 2

Plastic Governmentality

In November 2008, the Brazilian Federal Senate celebrated the sixtieth anniversary of the Brazilian Society of Plastic Surgery by holding a special session to pay homage to the medical specialty. Several senators expounded on the charitable work that had been done by plastic surgeons since Ivo Pitanguy first rose to the occasion in the 1960s. One senator even remarked upon the growth of plastic surgery in public hospitals, lauding the "fact" that, "nowadays, plastic surgery is more focused on the recovery of victims of accidents and disfigurements, than on aesthetic surgery."[1] The growth in the total number of plastic surgeries, therefore, had not gone unnoticed by government actors, but it was presumed to represent a growth in real need among the poorest members of the Brazilian population, not a growth in the number of aesthetic surgeries subsidized by the state. The national pride associated today with plastic surgery arises from the perception of plastic surgeons as great humanitarians who provide an irreplaceable service. As Brazil is transformed into a global center of knowledge about plastic surgery, attracting hundreds of foreign surgeons from around the world, the advances of the medical specialty become increasingly tied to nationalist narratives of progress. Today, criticizing the discipline of plastic surgery, particularly its place within public health, is paramount to criticizing the nation itself. Despite the very limited resources of the public health-care system, there are no detractors, or ethical discussions about the practice, in the Brazilian public sphere.

Plastic surgery established itself as a national biopolitical project that captures the imagination of actors across the spectrum of Brazilian society by performing what Bruno Latour describes as "lashing in" allies within networks. Latour suggests we should be skeptical of the facts produced by scientific and technological discourses, and that we should instead aim to describe how scientific alliances and knowledge production come into being through active social processes.[2] What follows is a portrait of plastic surgeons in action as they navigate the networks of Brazilian health care to recruit the state as an unwitting ally. I trace the ways by which plastic surgeons become fused with the state at specific junctures, or nodes, within the networks of public health care, appropriating the state's biopolitical authority for themselves. Plastic surgeons deploy a type of governance that I call "plastic governmentality"—a flexible approach to the management of public health that allows them to conceal its imbrication with commercial medicine. This flexibility makes it possible for plastic surgeons to bend hospital rules, relabel surgeries, and adjust waiting queues according to their own interests, yet to always present themselves as humanitarians providing a health service on behalf of the state, thus realigning national interests to match their own.

HYBRID MEDICINE

The Brazilian health-care system was marked by disparities in access and quality during a large part of the twentieth century. The sanitation movement led by the Oswaldo Cruz Institute from 1900 to 1930 was the first attempt at creating a state health policy, but its main aim was the eradication of disease through vaccines and hygienic education, not the construction of public hospitals. Those who could not afford the care of a private, university-trained doctor, depended on medical care provided by philanthropic hospitals managed by Christian brotherhoods, like the network of Santa Casa da Misericórdia hospitals founded under Portuguese colonial rule.[3] After Brazilian independence, these philanthropic hospitals received public funds to make necessary reforms and conform to modern standards of hygiene. They fell into disrepute among the working class, however, who rightfully saw them as way stations on the path to death and who preferred, whenever possible, to continue making use of practitioners of popular forms of medicine, such as herbalists, barber-surgeons, midwives, and *curandeiros* (healers).[4]

The Getúlio Vargas government (1930–1945) established the first social security system in Brazil with the creation of the Pensions and

Retirement Institutes (Institutos de Aposentadorias e Pensões), in which a worker was given access to a particular network of medical services through his or her affiliation with a given professional class.[5] This semi-iautonomous social security system was considered a government compromise in response to the demands of urban workers' unions, but it reinforced health disparities by providing better health coverage to professional classes with higher incomes, because they could afford to make higher monthly contributions to their given institutes and even establish their own hospitals. The system also excluded anyone who did not receive a regular salary, such as rural workers, the unemployed, and those who made a living from the informal economy.[6]

It was only in 1966, during the military dictatorship, that all the different pension and retirement programs were unified into a single government agency, the National Institute of Social Security (Instituto Nacional de Previdência Social, or INPS). Although it established the state as a centralized administrator of health services, this unification did not represent a significant expansion of the network of public hospitals. All salaried workers who paid a monthly contribution were integrated into the system, which increased the demand for services and forced the INPS to purchase medical services from private hospitals to complement its own health-care capabilities.[7] Private hospitals were remunerated according to a price chart that allocated a given sum per medical service, known as the units of service (unidades de serviço). There is evidence that many workers pushed for the use of private services owing to the ill repute of philanthropic and public hospitals, which were considered low-quality, charitable services for the indigent.[8]

In practice, this resulted in the rapid expansion, during the 1970s, of the private health-care system in Brazil, paid for with public social security funds, as more and more private hospitals vied to become accredited service providers for the INPS. It also promoted corruption, generated more expensive procedures, and stimulated the creation of many new private hospitals and medical schools that privileged specialized, profitable technologies rather than basic health care. During the military dictatorship, the health of the poorest Brazilians steadily deteriorated as unsalaried workers remained excluded from the social security system, and medical care for the poor was mostly limited to the Ministry of Health's combat and prevention of transmissible diseases in order to protect the rest of the population.[9]

The "economic miracle" of the 1970s, which saw the Brazilian economy grow astronomically even as social inequalities became exacerbated, provided the military government with increased revenue to fund the expanding private health-care system. During this decade, nearly 90 percent of all INPS expenses derived from the purchase of services from private medical providers, who conducted a large majority of all medical procedures.[10] By the 1980s, however, as the Brazilian economy entered a sharp downturn, it became clear that the funding of health-care services through the INPS was in crisis, making the current system untenable. Direct government subsidies were replaced with tax breaks for companies that continued to provide medical insurance to their employees, causing exponential growth in private insurance companies. The dictatorship's repressive measures weakened with the onset of the economic crisis, inaugurating a transitional period known as the "political opening" (*abertura política*), which allowed a growing number of social movements to push for a return to democracy in the country.

Within the area of health care, an alliance of medical students, doctors, and health officials formed the movement for Sanitation Reform (Reforma Sanitária), whose position was that only a universal health-care system would truly address the collective needs of Brazilian society. Their efforts won the inclusion of health care as a "right of all and an obligation of the state" in the new Brazilian constitution of 1988, and a commitment from the newly democratic government to significantly expand and decentralize the public health-care system.[11] The movement's most radical proposal, however, which entailed nationalizing all medical care, fell by the wayside with the organized opposition of a now powerful private hospital industry. There was also a lack of support from the middle class and workers' unions, which saw private insurance and private medical providers as more reliable.[12] The basic right to health care, therefore, remained subordinate to the right of private medical providers to sell health as a consumer item.

The political project of giving equitable health care to all Brazilians remained unrealized, then, as public health care was reinscribed as a resource for the neediest but not an entitlement of society as a whole. The Unified Health System (Sistema Único de Saúde, or SUS), as the Brazilian universal health-care system came to be known, has consistently suffered from underfunding and, even today, lacks a secure source of financial support to guarantee its operations.[13] The problems of the SUS are a political liability to governmental social policies, as it has become easy for political opponents, in criticizing current administrations, to point out its failures rather than its merits. Similarly, providers of private insurance plans criticize the deficiencies of the SUS as a marketing strategy to capture more clients. The disrepute of the universal health-care system remains strong in the mainstream media, even though many national health indicators have significantly improved since it was implemented.[14]

More importantly for my argument, the public health-care system remains what I call, following Telma Menucucci, a "hybrid" structure, whereby a large amount of public funding needs to be funneled through private hospitals in order to reach the general population. According to the most recent statistics supplied by the Brazilian Federation of Hospitals, more than 40 percent of private hospitals have contractual agreements with the state to provide medical services for the SUS. This figure is not surprising by itself, until we take into account the fact that the private sector is now responsible for 62 percent of all medical procedures the SUS carries out.[15] In other words, the state still heavily depends on subcontracting privately owned hospitals to complement its own medical services, although to a lesser extent than before. This hybridity allows the private medical care industry to keep growing, since its source of income remains flexible and comes from both private insurance and the SUS.

The aim of the Brazilian health-care system, then, is to provide universal access to Brazilian citizens, but the production of medical services remains highly privatized and hardly universal. Rather than being evenly distributed across the population, most of the private medical resources are amassed and used in the richest regions and cities in the country, reinforcing the health disparities in Brazil. Many critics of the ongoing reliance of the SUS on private health care have described it as acquiescing to the neoliberal ideology that seeks to reduce the participation of the state in the economy. Although universal health care was instituted in 1988, the Brazilian governments of the 1990s strongly favored privatizing rather than expanding public services, influenced by the free-market agenda promoted by global lending institutions like the World Bank and the International Monetary Fund. It is surprising, however, that this neoliberal logic continued to have a strong hold during the administration of the Workers' Party, which some academics described as a "postneoliberal" moment in Brazilian history.[16] Despite a call to strengthen the welfare state, neoliberal governmentality remained a standard characteristic of many of the state's operations, particularly the mixed public/private approach to health care.

This produced a contradiction within the politics of public health, where the effort to give more people access to health care was tempered by the aim to foster the participation of the private health sector. In other words, publicly funded health care expanded primarily by means of private mechanisms. As Aihwa Ong has demonstrated, neoliberal governmentality takes diverse forms, and some of its iterations do not seek to dismantle the welfare state but, rather, deploy it to benefit private interests.[17] Moreover, any gains in social services are likely to be reversed when neoliberal governments implement austerity programs. The current government, which took control after the controversial impeachment of Dilma Rousseff, has used Brazil's economic crisis as an excuse to severely cut funding for public health, putting at risk the very stability of the whole SUS.[18]

The case of Brazilian health care is important because it represents an exception to the standard narrative about the neoliberal shift within contemporary biopolitics. In this narrative, today's "politics of life itself" is marked by a reduction of the state's role in the management of health, replaced by a new political rationality that emphasizes nonstate regulatory mechanisms and the responsibility of consumer-citizens to pay for their own health care.[19] In Brazil, it is paradoxically the state expansion of public health that has produced new hybrid forms of governance that are neither purely public nor capable of existing independently of the state. The expansion of plastic surgery within the public health-care system depends directly on these technologies of governance that deploy the welfare state to strengthen private ventures. Plastic surgery patients, in this scenario, are interstitial actors caught between the public and the private, negotiating their health needs simultaneously as citizen demands and as consumer desires. Plastic surgeons, on the other hand, are hybrid actors with dual allegiances, given that they act as "gatekeepers" for the state, deciding how to allocate resources and favoring procedures that generate profit within the private market. The plastic surgeries taking place in publicly funded Brazilian hospitals, therefore, articulate the blurred borderlands between public health and commercial medicine.

THE "PITANGUYNIZATION" OF BRAZIL

At the Ivo Pitanguy Institute in Rio de Janeiro, the lines begin to form at five in the morning, even though the doors will not open for another two hours. The patients hope their early arrival will guarantee their spot in the series of interviews, medical examinations, and psychological evaluations that are prerequisites to the low-cost plastic surgery the institute offers. Almost all the patients who frequent the institute are working-class; and although these surgeries cost a fifth of what they

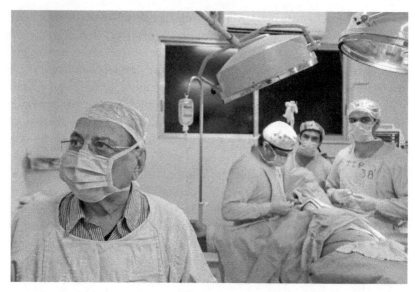

FIG 5. Ivo Pitanguy monitoring a surgery performed by medical residents at the Santa Casa da Misericórdia. Photo courtesy of Vincent Rosenblatt.

would cost in a private clinic, they represent a sizable share of the patients' incomes. Many of the patients comment that they have been saving for months or years for their surgery at this reputable institute.

The Ivo Pitanguy Institute is located in a renovated wing of the Santa Casa da Misericórdia, an old philanthropic Catholic hospital founded in the colonial period, known for being chronically underfunded and having severe infrastructure problems. The institute stands out as the hospital's one redeeming quality, however, since it bears the name of the most famous plastic surgeon in Brazilian history, considered a great humanitarian and a symbol of Brazilian medical progress. Before his death in 2016, Pitanguy won several national and international distinctions "for his work with less-favored populations."[20] He has become a living myth in Brazilian popular culture, and his name is recognized internationally among plastic surgeons, who consider his institute to be one of the most important learning institutions in the world. The Ivo Pitanguy Institute thus not only provides beauty for the poor in Brazil but is also an educational center that trains surgeons and produces medical knowledge that circulates globally (see fig. 5).

According to the institute's own estimates, nearly forty-four thousand low-income patients have undergone operations here since it was first founded in 1960, an average of more than a thousand patients a year. By 2003, it had fully educated 448 plastic surgeons from thirty-six different countries and had provided briefer training to nearly four thousand other surgeons.[21] Most importantly, the medical residency program at the Ivo Pitanguy Institute has become the educational model followed by most other medical institutions in Brazil that specialize in plastic surgery, particularly in metropolitan areas of the wealthier Brazilian Southeast. Since the creation of a Brazilian universal health-care system in 1988, plastic surgery residency programs in publicly funded hospitals have been provided with state resources to maintain and expand their operations. Many of those residency programs are led by former students of the Ivo Pitanguy Institute, who defend plastic surgery as an essential humanitarian service that should be made available to patients of all backgrounds. As I see it, there is an underlying contradiction between the alleged humanitarian nature of their work, and the stipulation that poor patients must be willing to become experimental subjects to have access to beauty. The national and international credibility of the profession, however, is directly linked to the simultaneous representation of plastic surgery in publicly funded hospitals as philanthropic and as productive of medical knowledge.

The central conceit of plastic surgery's illustrious national reputation is the variable deployment of the practice's two subdisciplines: aesthetic surgery and reconstructive surgery. On the one hand, plastic surgeons make a distinction between the aesthetic procedures provided to private consumers and the reconstructive surgeries made available to the poor in public hospitals. In the public imagination, reconstructive surgeries are associated with plastic surgeons' charitable work for the poor: surgeries that treat accidental injuries, burns, and congenital deformities. In practice, however, the difference between the aesthetic and reconstructive categories is actively blurred by plastic surgeons, who depend on this synthesis in order to facilitate the transfer of knowledge from publicly funded hospitals, where clinical studies take place, to their more lucrative private practices. Moreover, plastic surgeons describe aesthetic surgeries to their low-income patients as exceptional favors they will generously perform out of kindness, summoning the gratitude of these patients even as the patients agree to become subjects for clinical study. In order to make the aesthetic/reconstructive conceit possible, plastic surgeons must recruit the Brazilian state itself as an ally, because the state is the main source of funding for reconstructive procedures. This alliance was forged over the course of several decades, based on the slow expansion of the definition of *reconstructive* to include an increasing number of plastic surgeries. Today, plastic surgery is a national hallmark of Brazilian public medicine, but that was not the case seventy years ago.

According to Ivo Pitanguy's autobiography, *The Right to Beauty*, when he began practicing medicine in 1949 he had to work very hard at convincing his colleagues that plastic surgery was a medical specialty that had a place in publicly funded hospitals. They were initially hostile to the idea and claimed that he "was using that mass of poor people as 'guinea pigs' and . . . taking advantage of them to 'make [his] hand,' an unfair expression they used back then."[22] The phrase "make his hand" referred to the surgical dexterity and clinical knowledge that Pitanguy was gaining by having access to these new patients. Owing to the dearth of medical schools that provided training in plastic surgery in Brazil, Pitanguy had studied the discipline in the United States and Europe, with plastic surgeons renowned for their work in reconstructing the disfigured faces of soldiers from the two world wars. In order to gain support for his practice, Pitanguy contended that Brazil might not have had victims of war, but it had very similar conditions in the violence of its favelas: "The experiences I had as I explored the alleyways of favelas, and during my stay in the United States, when I witnessed the return of mutilated soldiers with disfigured faces, made evident that suffering is the same in all latitudes and hemispheres. . . . We live in an era of permanent trauma. Even if war creates a greater concentration of it, the day-to-day succession of urban violence creates just as many mutilations as war."[23] By associating urban violence with war, Pitanguy tapped into the Brazilian imaginary about crime and disorder in the favelas and the fear that this violence might spill out into middle-class neighborhoods. If narratives of violence undergird the logic of beautification in Brazil, it is because ugliness is a symbol of social disorder and Brazil's stark social inequalities. Plastic surgery is imagined as capable of stitching bodies back together and dispelling those inequalities, providing an invaluable service to the nation.

The 1950s and 1960s witnessed rapid urbanization in Brazil, in which large numbers of poor rural workers migrated to urban areas in search of work.[24] Most of them settled in favelas, the shantytowns that, over decades, had slowly spread on the hillsides around cities like Rio de Janeiro, but which had grown exponentially during this period. Brazilian newspapers from this era were filled with accounts of criminals— frequently described by the darkness of their skin and their "ugliness"— descending from the hillsides to attack "innocent" residents of wealthier areas. Pitanguy capitalized on this fear by claiming that plastic surgery repaired not only accidental mutilations but also congenital deformities that might alter a person's character. He made the case that the correction of deformities through plastic surgery could help reintegrate the favela's social misfits into society, absolving the upper-middle class from the economic and political forms of exclusion it perpetrated on the poor, stating, "Physical defects influence the human being in such a way that anthropological studies done on incarcerated criminals show significant behavior changes in those whose undesirable features, which differentiated them from others, were corrected."[25]

Pitanguy resurrected old arguments from criminology to present his work in public hospitals as a form of humanitarian service that could improve not only the lives of individuals but the whole of society as well. The specter of the natural-born criminal, identifiable through his physical appearance, could be resolved by excising those undesirable physical features. The normalization of these patients through surgery was imagined as removing the racialized traits of their poverty. Thus, Pitanguy reinforced the association between beautification and the betterment of society, supplying plastic surgery with a basis for its expansion in public hospitals. His appeals won him the backing of then-President Kubitschek, who in 1960 provided Pitanguy with funding to open a plastic surgery service for the poor, which would double as a medical school, at the Santa Casa da Misericórdia. This service was framed as completely different from the service provided by Pitanguy to wealthier clients in his upscale, private clinic located in a middle-class neighborhood of Rio de Janeiro.

What catapulted Ivo Pitanguy to national fame was, not surprisingly, one of these scenes of criminal violence, whose tragic proportions helped cement it in collective memory. When I asked my interviewees what they had first heard about Pitanguy, most recalled his role in helping the victims of the fire that had occurred during a circus performance in the middle-class neighborhood of Niterói in Rio de Janeiro, on December 1961. The tragedy resulted in nearly five hundred deaths and more than twenty-five hundred injured survivors, many of them children with severe burns, which prompted the mobilization of many doctors, including Pitanguy and his team. Journalistic accounts of the time focused not only on the efforts to help the victims but also on the police investigation into the cause of the fire. Despite reports that three other tents of the same circus had burned down on previous occasions owing to faulty electrical wiring, suspicion quickly fell on a "dark-skinned 19-year-old man" with a history of psychiatric problems, and on other "*favelados* [people from the favelas] who had caused disturbances" after proprietors denied them entrance to the circus.[26] The investigators concluded these *favelados* had set fire to the circus in revenge for their humiliation. An editorial described the perpetrators as "not having a conscience," and went on to say, about criminals in general: "They act out of beastly instinct . . . and are a product of the environment they grow up in, in the margins of society. These *marginais* [criminals] are being produced by the thousands in front of our eyes."[27]

In contrast to this depiction of a wild, senseless criminality coming from the favelas, plastic surgeons were portrayed as restoring order by caring for the victims and repairing their scarred bodies. Pitanguy gained special recognition for getting the U.S. government to donate three hundred square meters of freeze-dried human skin to graft onto the burn victims.[28] Not only was this a marvel of modern American technology transplanted onto Brazilian bodies, but it also seemed to provide solace to the victims of the tragic crime that had been committed. It was as if the imported skin, imagined as white, could effectively reverse the violence associated with darker skin.

The circus tragedy is a narrative still recounted to this day, always in association with Pitanguy, and it has provided him with the moral authority to claim that the absence of beauty is a serious medical and ethical problem that should be addressed by plastic surgeons. In the introduction to *The Right to Beauty*, Ivo Pitanguy uses his recollections about the circus burn victims he cared for to argue that aesthetic surgery is as crucial as reconstructive surgery: "Sometimes it was almost unbearable to see certain victims, made monstrous by the fire. Could I be satisfied with keeping them alive, now that the horrible scars embedded in their faces or their bodies would transform their lives into permanent torment? . . . Could it be possible that surgery could content itself with repairing? Would it be normal to simply think about preserving a life and ignore the beauty of a face?"[29] It was his experience with the circus tragedy, Pitanguy argues, that convinced him to fight against ugliness itself and to combine aesthetic and reconstructive surgery into a single practice.

The title of Pitanguy's autobiography summarizes his view that beauty is an essential aspect of health care, and that it should be provided by both public and private hospitals. Even today, plastic surgeons and their patients in the public health-care system use the term *right to beauty* to explain why plastic surgery should be accessible to everyone. Pitanguy thus laid the groundwork for blurring the distinction between reconstructive and aesthetic surgeries, making it easier for surgeons, medical residents, and patients to rebrand elective medical procedures as medically indispensable. If the rise and respectability of Brazilian plastic surgery is synonymous with Ivo Pitanguy, it is because his name is a signifier not just for his practice but also for the educational format that gives plastic surgery its humanitarian image.

COSMETIC RECONSTRUCTIONS

Every Thursday at Rio de Janeiro's First Federal Hospital, the plastic surgery team gathered at the hospital's top floor, where they would change into scrubs and enter the operating rooms for that week's scheduled surgeries. I had been frequenting this public hospital for several weeks, invited by the chief plastic surgeon, Dr. Mario, who owned a private clinic in a wealthy neighborhood of Rio but taught here at the hospital. He treated me like the first-year medical residents, allowing me to observe the consultations, surgeries, and postoperative care involving plastic surgery patients. On this particular Thursday, Dr. Mario and I sat in the coffee room, taking a break from surgery while the rest of the team toiled away in the operating rooms. I asked Dr. Mario why he thought there were so many aesthetic surgeries in Brazil. He responded, "Everyone wonders why there is so much [aesthetic] plastic surgery in Brazil, but that is because they believe Brazil is all African and poor. In reality, there are two Brazils: the Brazil that is poor and miserable, and the Brazil that is rich and developed. As Delfim Netto [former minister of finance] said, Brazil is a BelIndia, half Belgium, half India. The developed Brazil wants plastic surgery because we live in a world of competition, where image is given a lot of importance. The other half of Brazil is indeed African and Asiatic."[30]

His answer surprised me, not only because it seemed to pigeonhole aesthetic surgery as a consumer desire exclusively of a whiter and wealthier population, but also because it negated all the aesthetic surgeries occurring at that very moment in the operating rooms less than a hundred feet from where we sat. I asked Dr. Mario to explain why, then, so many aesthetic surgeries were undertaken at public hospitals like this one. He answered that performing aesthetic surgery in public hospitals had "become a necessity" owing to the large number of doctors training to be plastic surgeons and the high demand from society for this kind of surgery. This was, however, simply "an anomaly, a distortion permitted by the hospital structure."

For Dr. Mario, the growth of aesthetic surgery in public hospitals is a distortion because aesthetic surgery would always be, in his eyes, a practice of the rich and developed Brazil and thus firmly located within private health care. Many other plastic surgeons I interviewed also argued that their medical specialty is a symbol of the country's development, as the most cutting-edge medical specialty in the country. As such, its appropriate setting is the luxurious consultation room and impeccable private clinic, where the upper-middle class purchases aesthetic surgery, not the rundown public hospital. Instead, the surgeries that should ideally be carried out in public hospitals are reconstructive surgeries, whose main purpose is not to beautify but to address a medical ailment and restore a body's normal function.

According to Dr. Mario, however, it was becoming increasingly difficult to differentiate between the reconstructive and aesthetic categories, because almost any surgery could be described as restoring health rather than enhancing a body, echoing the claims first made by Ivo Pitanguy. The only clear distinction between aesthetic and reconstructive surgeries, therefore, is the setting where they take place and the bodies that they act upon. The poor patients who seek care at publicly funded hospitals are construed as a population entirely distinct from the patients at a plastic surgeon's private practice—distinct not only because of their social class but also because of their imagined "African and Asiatic" racial difference. Since residency programs are located in publicly funded hospitals, the bodies of these patients are considered the most suitable for plastic surgeons in training to learn their trade on.

The Brazilian medical establishment, therefore, establishes a hidden contract similar to the one described by Foucault in *The Birth of the Clinic,* where treatment is given to the poor in exchange for their presence as objects of clinical observation in order to train doctors.[31] The medical knowledge that is most valued in this exchange in Brazil is the knowledge that translates into profit in the private market. The medical residents I interviewed understood reconstructive surgeries for burn victims and surgeries to correct congenital deformities as bothersome chores from which they could learn very little. They valued instead the surgeries most desired by their potential private customers, such as breast lifts and nose surgeries.

The aesthetic surgeries performed in publicly funded hospitals that Dr. Mario portrays as anomalies, therefore, have become the keystone for plastic surgery training in Brazil. The unease or outright disavowal that Dr. Mario and other surgeons expressed in relation to these surgeries arises from how this practice contradicts the public perception of their profession. Admitting that these surgeries are central to building their own knowledge and reputation would put into question the neat separation between public and private health, and it would problematize the notion that aesthetic surgery is aligned with medical modernity and the rich citizens of developed Brazil. Furthermore, Brazilian law states that only reconstructive surgery can be paid for with public funds. The aesthetic surgeries conducted in publicly funded hospitals have to relabeled as reconstructive surgeries in order to get the state to fund them. This renaming is an everyday practice that most plastic surgery residents perform unthinkingly and is thus a central aspect of plastic governmentality.

Another ethnographic scene that took place at First Federal Hospital illustrates how renaming surgeries alters state perceptions about the practice. One Thursday, I was observing a face-lift procedure in an operating room, dressed in scrubs and taking field notes. The surgery was conducted by third-year residents and watched attentively by other students, for whom a face-lift was a special treat that did not occur often. They had made the case that they needed to be proficient in aesthetic surgery so that when they opened their own private practices, they would not commit errors and get sued by their wealthier patients. This was not just any face-lift either: it was a mini-lipo-face-lift, which removes excess fat from the face at the same time that it reduces wrinkles, and it had been one of the most interesting novelties presented at the last national plastic surgery conference. Dr. Mario had approved his students' involvement in the procedure so they could try it out for the first time and evaluate its advantages and drawbacks.

At the end of the operation, as the patient slowly awakened, Dr. Mario told a second-year resident who was filling out the forms to record the surgery as a correction of facial paralysis. The resident asked why they could not admit that the surgery was a face-lift, given that everyone knows that all public hospitals perform these surgeries. Dr. Mario gave her a stern look and reminded her that the official position of the Brazilian Society of Plastic Surgery is that aesthetic surgery occurs only in private clinics. An innovative aesthetic procedure that is valuable to residents, therefore, becomes a reconstructive procedure on the only hospital form that the state will have access to when producing national statistics. What doctors choose to see and register in public hospitals determines what the government officially perceives as well. Within spaces such as consultation offices and operating rooms, where knowledge is as transient as the bodies moving through them, doctors and residents *are* the state while simultaneously representing private interests that exceed the aims of the state.

THE PLASTICITY OF NUMBERS

Recall the ceremony in which the Brazilian Senate celebrated plastic surgery as a form of patrimony that had made indelible contributions to the nation. Senators asserted that plastic surgery was increasingly concerned with reconstructive surgeries, because this is the information that the official statistics provide—reconstructive surgeries in publicly funded hospitals are on the rise across Brazil, numbering in the hundreds of thousands each year. From the point of view of the Brazilian government, these surgeries are completely justified public health expenses, because in the public imaginary they represent mostly burn victims, people with congenital deformities, and victims of violence. This is the type of charitable work that made Ivo Pitanguy famous; it is not public knowledge that 95 percent of the surgeries carried out at the Santa Casa are purely aesthetic.

The mainstream media reiterates these narratives: an article in the influential *Veja* magazine remarked on the fact that in the span of a decade, reconstructive procedures had increased nearly tenfold. The cause for this increase was portrayed as an increase in criminal violence, where plastic surgeons have had to repair "severed fingers and ears, stomachs punctured by bullet wounds or cut open by knives . . . [and] faces disfigured by violent punches." In the same article, the president of the Brazilian Society of Plastic Surgery lamented this trend, declaring, "Violence in Brazil has reached a level that alters even our national statistics."[32] Altered statistics about plastic surgery evoke fear because they are imagined as an index of urban violence, and the role of plastic surgeons in public hospitals is assumed to be one in which they suture the wounds of the body politic and reshape the features of society.

Statistics are powerful symbols because, as James Scott argues, they can be deployed to give meaning to events and trends at the same time that they simplify our view of the world by reducing complex realities to myopic standardized measurements.[33] I argue, however, that governance sometimes *relies* on complex realities remaining illegible to civil society and even the state itself. Plastic governmentality, in particular, is abetted by official statistics that do not merely distort reality but interact with the state to produce the very state practices and policies that these numbers describe.

According to Claudia Travassos, a public researcher for the Fiocruz Institute who has analyzed the reliability of the SUS, this system—and the perhaps the state in its entirety—can be understood as little more than a system of resource allocation and the collection of statistics.[34] Based on the structure set up during the 1970s for social security, the SUS continues to provide payments to individual medical providers according to a table that establishes a standard price for a given medical procedure. Each hospital produces the statistics for its own operations, which means that the statistical inflation of or undernotification about certain medical treatments is a somewhat common occurrence. The government usually responds to patients' complaints about inadequate treatment in the public health-care system by injecting more funding into it, but not by increasing the oversight of how the funding is used. Thus, the statistics on the growing number of plastic surgeries paid for by the public health-care system seem to verify that plastic surgery addresses real medical needs of the working-class Brazilian population and work to provide justification for approving additional funding for it. As Diane Nelson argues, accounting and mathematics are a form of politics by other means, and numbers can become situated nonhuman agents that enable particular forms of power relations.[35]

Additionally, plastic surgery statistics are used to justify an increase in the types of procedures permitted under the federal guidelines. In Brazil, the Federal Council of Medicine (Conselho Federal de Medicina, or CFM)—an institution that possesses the legal authority to assess, regulate, and standardize all medical activities in the country—determines the guidelines for deciding which procedures should be covered by the state. The CFM's technical commissions for each medical specialty, which make rulings pertaining to issues relevant to that specialty, are composed of doctors indirectly chosen by their peers. Thus, the council's technical commission for plastic surgery is entirely composed of plastic surgeons, most of whom also act as professors for medical residency programs. The resolutions and rulings of technical commissions, if approved by the CFM board, have the force of law, and the Ministry of Health usually adopts these rulings as the norms to be used within each medical specialty in the context of the universal health-care system. The technical commission for plastic surgery has pushed for designating a wide variety of plastic surgeries as reconstructive surgeries and, therefore, for letting the public health-care system cover their costs.

For example, in 2003 the CFM ruled that reduction mastoplasties and abdominal dermolipectomies, commonly known in English as breast reductions and tummy tucks, should be considered nonaesthetic surgeries when excess breast or abdominal tissue is causing a patient back pain.[36] The ruling quotes Pitanguy's studies of those medical conditions, using his authority as the main reasoning behind the ruling. Even though these surgeries had been taking place in some public hospitals for more than a decade, the ruling made the practice official for all public hospitals. Two important aspects of this and other resolutions is that they unequivocally state that patients' requests for reconstructive surgery are on the rise, and they argue that there should be rigorous scientific criteria to determine whether a surgery is reconstructive or aesthetic, without ever specifying what those criteria might be. Thus, the expansion of the reconstructive category is portrayed as arising from patient demand, not from surgeons' demands. Moreover, there are no clear national standards for diagnosing whether a surgery is aesthetic or reconstructive, and the decision is thus delegated to surgeons themselves.

Today, tummy tucks and breast reductions are two of the most common surgeries that take place in publicly funded hospitals, but plastic surgeons do not require a medical exam to corroborate a patient's claim of back pain. When I was present during consultations, it became clear that surgeons asked suggestive questions to prompt the patient to express his or her physical discomfort. Many patients in the waiting room coached other patients on the "correct" things to say and symptoms to exhibit in order to have their surgery approved. I witnessed several instances where female patients had no trouble with the size of their breasts but were bothered instead by their flaccidness. These patients got medical approval for a breast reduction, but the actual surgery they received would be more accurately described as a breast lift, since no breast tissue was removed. Similarly, nose jobs (rhinoplasties) are routinely described as the correction of a deviated septum, eyelid surgeries (blepharoplasties) are justified as improving a patient's eyesight, and vaginal rejuvenations (ninfoplasties or labiaplasties) become reconstructive surgeries to fix anomalous genitalia. Once a given reconstructive surgery is approved, the topography of the body that the surgery targets is made available not for one but for a series of medical interventions. There was a gendered aspect to these interventions as well: many more surgeries were routinely approved for women's bodies, and the medical knowledge regarding women's bodies was perceived as more valuable by residents (see fig. 6).

According to government data on the SUS, however, 100 percent of the plastic surgeries occurring through this system are reconstructive surgeries. Dr. Paulo, a member of the statistical department at the Ministry of Health, offered a plausible explanation for why the aesthetic surgeries I had ethnographically observed remained invisible to the state: the series of available databases on the public health-care system

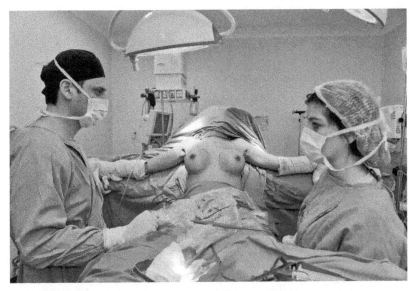

FIG 6. Medical residents verifying that breast implants are even after performing surgery at a publicly funded hospital. Photo courtesy of Vincent Rosenblatt.

does not even consider aesthetic surgeries as valid values to be entered. Only reconstructive surgeries have their own categories and corresponding codes within the long list of permitted medical procedures, from which surgeons choose when they are filling out the forms after each operation. Dr. Paulo explained that data used to be more accurate a decade ago, when surgeons had to write in their own diagnoses rather than choose from a list. As the system of gathering data becomes more modernized and automated, more information is lost, because surgeons simply look for the codified categories that most closely resemble the procedures they carry out.

Dr. Paulo still believed, however, that surgeons are trustworthy gate-keepers for the allocation of public resources, because they understand local health needs that supersede national directives. Statistical inaccuracies reflected errors in data collection, not in the health-care system itself. Thus, the norms and regulations of the public health-care system are understood as a flexible blueprint that becomes imbricated with informal arrangements specific to each locality. Dr. Paulo acknowledged that he was aware that aesthetic surgeries indeed occurred that were covered by public funds, since he had an aunt who had gotten a nose job at a public hospital. Yet he suggested that bringing this fact to the public's attention could hinder the efforts of patients who truly deserved reconstructive surgery through the public health-care system at one hospital or another.

SURGERIES WITH JEITINHO

Michel Foucault defines governmentality as the institutions, procedures, and analyses that allow the modern administrative state to manage economies and populations. The tactics of government, he argues, have become dispersed throughout society, enlisting individuals to discipline, optimize, and regulate each other in relation to an imagined greater good, transforming the state into a "composite reality and a mythicised abstraction."[37] As Diane Nelson argues, however, this abstraction still produces awe, fear, and hate precisely because it is not a "one-way activity of the state on the people" but rather a "state-effect [that] emerges from . . . multiplicities of exchanges" involving the collaboration of every actor within society.[38] The state comes into being, in other words, through the constant circulation of social activities linked to its imaginary presence, whereby the state is nowhere and everywhere at the same time. At times the state may appear to be a willfully duplicitous power, Nelson cautions, yet it functions only through our coparticipation as state subjects, its two-facedness a mirror of our own.

When the Brazilian state relies on hybrid public-private mechanisms to distribute public resources, it is not necessarily being duplicitous about its objective to distribute health care more equitably, but it is recruited to participate in privatized networks that prioritize profit-generating procedures. Public health is experienced as a diverse collection of institutions with sometimes overlapping and sometimes contradictory aims. Similarly, plastic surgeons who rename surgeries so that they correspond to permissible state diagnoses consider themselves not duplicitous but true to the needs of the medical residents who make plastic surgery in publicly funded hospitals possible in the first place. Through their expertise, plastic surgeons transform the "right to beauty" into a hybrid application of aesthetic and reconstructive surgery, attracting the widespread support of civil society.

What I call plastic governmentality, therefore, can be defined as the pliability of the state itself in the service of statecraft as it bends to accommodate the myriad interests that invoke the state as their interlocutor. I believe neoliberal governmentality depends more on this pliability than did previous forms of governance, because it instrumentalizes government operations in favor of private interests. The state becomes a guarantor for unofficial practices that exceed the state's own explicit aims, but which benefit hybrid actors that represent themselves as allies to the state. Plastic surgeons' claims that they are performing humanitarian work lashes in the state by invoking the state's explicit aim to provide basic health care to all its citizens. The highly publicized cases of burn victims being treated and disfigured patients being healed stand in for all the surgeries performed on the poor in public hospitals. Thus, surgeons transform their own vision of the public health-care system into the state's vision, providing themselves with leeway to circumvent or even shape the state's policies and regulations while gaining prestige. This prestige depends on a form of accounting that is also pliable, producing official figures regarding reconstructive surgery that reinforce the practice.

Likewise, patients in publicly funded hospitals are aware that the aesthetic surgeries they are offered depend on plastic surgeons bending the rules, and they actively collaborate to make that happen. They describe the understanding between patients and surgeons that permits the circumvention of official norms as being able to *dar um jeitinho,* or "provide a way" to get the surgeries approved by the state. The anthropologist Roberto DaMatta describes *jeitinho* as a Brazilian cultural practice involving an informal arrangement between a common individual making a request and a person in position of authority. The *jeitinho* finds a creative solution to a bureaucratic impasse, whereby the authority makes an exception and allows the petitioner to forgo some of the requirements usually associated with the request. The social reality, therefore, transcends the impersonal force of law, which most Brazilians consider to be imperfect and inapplicable as a universal.[39] More recently, Livia Barbosa has described the *jeitinho* as a mechanism of power within Brazilian society that has an important symbolic value, because it is ultimately a narrative about Brazilian national character that legitimizes differential treatment under the law. *Jeitinho* is a predictable narrative interpreted by working-class actors, in particular, as a means to humanize the law in a way that benefits them.[40] Given the inequalities historically written into Brazilian law to exclude the dispossessed,[41] the *jeitinho* is predominantly understood as an extralegal practice that nonetheless democratizes access.

Plastic governmentality is particularly successful in Brazil because it relies on this social expectation that the bureaucracy will permit certain exceptions. When surgeons justify aesthetic surgeries for their patients in publicly funded hospitals, these patients interpret it as a *jeitinho* that remedies the bureaucratic imperfections of the public health-care system. In many cases, having a personal connection with a surgeon who works in a publicly funded hospital can effectively prioritize one's name in the long waiting list and shorten the time before surgery. At the hospitals where I conducted research, it was common for plastic surgeons to arrange surgeries for their employees and acquaintances, as a form of patronage that might complement payment for services. Even though these surgeries are made possible only through public funding, patients see them as facilitated by surgeons.

As Maria Antonia, a patient at the Ivo Pitanguy Institute, remarked, "While the government does not offer basic things, Pitanguy offers us the opportunity to be beautiful." In Maria Antonia's reasoning, Pitanguy (and all the plastic surgeons he metonymically represents) provides a service on behalf of a neglectful state, bestowing a benefit that would not otherwise become available. Plastic surgeries arranged through *jeitinho* thus garner recognition, admiration, and gratitude only for plastic surgeons, not for the hybrid medical system that makes those surgeries possible in the first place. The informal arrangement of providing aesthetic surgeries through *jeitinho* has become the unstated rule, rather than the exception, of surgical practice in the public health-care system. The *jeitinho* becomes an informal law that supersedes state regulations, making the exception an instrument of governmentality.

FORGOTTEN PATIENTS

The burn unit at Hospital das Cruzes, a small municipal hospital in Rio de Janeiro, is severely understaffed, despite the severity of the cases it treats and despite receiving patients from the entire state. At the time of my visit, every bed was occupied, and patients suffered from a wide variety of burns: two patients were homeless men who had been set on fire by drunk teenagers and nearly died, two men were laborers who had lost limbs after severe electrical burns, a woman had burns on her entire body from a car accident, a teenage girl was recovering from burns caused by a corrosive oil she had used while sunbathing, and a seven-year-old boy had extensive keloids on his skin from a household burning accident. All of these burns required different treatments, and Dr. Cecilia, the pediatrician who was running the unit, was barely able to keep up with the demands of her work.

Dr. Cecilia told me that despite never having specialized in burn care, she noticed the urgent needs in the area and had taught herself how to treat burn victims. The unit demanded all of her time, and she had very little support to run it. She had one plastic surgeon on staff, but he put more emphasis on his private practice and was frequently absent. She was also in urgent need of more expensive materials to treat the burns, such as a specialized mesh that could have easily prevented the keloids in the seven-year-old, but the hospital was chronically underfunded. Looking to raise additional resources through charity, Dr. Cecilia had created a foundation called the "Ivo Pitanguy Association to Support Burn Victims." She had not received any support from Ivo Pitanguy or anyone in his institute, but she hoped that Pitanguy's fame from treating burn victims would help her recruit donors.

The very procedures that make plastic surgery renowned as a medical practice in the public imaginary—such as the treatment of burn victims— are in reality the priority of very few doctors, and the patients who need them are found languishing in underfunded and understaffed hospitals, pushed out by the aesthetic procedures that are prioritized by plastic governmentality. A nurse who had worked for thirty years at the Ivo Pitanguy Institute in the Santa Casa assured me that this had not always been the case, and that reconstructive procedures had indeed been a priority when she began working there. Slowly, however, aesthetic procedures had begun taking more and more space in the Santa Casa, based on medical students' demands for knowledge. Patients are valued as experimental subjects only insofar as their surgeries have an aesthetic application outside the publicly funded hospital (the question of why and how they consent to become experimental subjects is covered in chapter 6).

If beauty is now considered a right in Brazil, it is one apportioned unequally, according to the informal norms established by plastic surgeons. As João Biehl points out, sometimes the people in greatest need in Brazil are made socially invisible by the same forms of biopolitical governance that were originally designed to care for them.[42] Plastic governmentality constructs a neoliberal biopolitical regime that instrumentalizes public health in the name of profit while accumulating symbolic capital for plastic surgeons for their "charitable" work on the poor. By fusing their own interests with those of the state, plastic surgeons have become icons of the cosmetic nation they founded. Once the doors to the public hospital close behind them, however, they take the "right to beauty" with them.

CHAPTER 3

The Circulation of Beauty

Amelia's voice broke and her eyes filled with tears when I asked her, in the waiting room of the Santa Casa, why she wanted a plastic surgery. After discovering cysts on her breasts, she had become extremely uncomfortable with their appearance and how they felt to the touch. Despite the diagnosis declaring these cysts benign and establishing that no surgery was medically necessary, she strongly desired plastic surgery to repair her body. Had the cysts compromised her health, she would have been able to have the operation without much delay, but the queues for free elective surgery in the public health-care system were nearly two years long. She had thus decided to spend her own money to pay for a low-cost surgery, which represented a very big expense for Amelia. She made a living as a maid and had had to scrape what she could from her meager earnings for a whole year before saving enough for the surgery.

The wealthy never faced the hardships she had to face, Amelia complained, adding:

> I believe that only those with money are able to operate a lot, it is much more difficult for a poor woman to become beautiful. . . . I do not find it cheap; I had to take money away from many other things. . . . I think it will lift my morale, and I will improve. I haven't been leaving my house except for work, and I am ashamed of going to the beach. It's as if I was *morta-viva* [(one of the) living dead]. I did not have the time to care of myself; I never went to the gym. . . . It's completely different for those who have the money: they can just go to the best plastic surgery clinics.

For Amelia, to be a poor woman without access to beauty was to be like the living dead, uncannily out of place in the world of the living. She described a powerful feeling of abjection produced by the inability to take care of herself, which shamed her and limited her ability to participate in society. She strongly believed plastic surgery would repair her body, giving her back a sense of bodily worth—beautification would make her someone who mattered again.

Amelia's narrative and her affective response capture very clearly the significance given to beauty by my Brazilian interviewees, especially those who were also members of the working class. They portrayed their desire for plastic surgery not as a vain impulse but as an absolute necessity for maintaining their social worth. Most of them described their surgeries as bodily repairs that were not merely aesthetic. Like Amelia, they contrasted their own difficulties in their pursuit of beauty to the ease with which the wealthy could acquire it. Beauty is something precarious and relational—it is in short supply, and it matters because it marks some bodies as having more money and leisure time than others, enabling them to frequent gyms, beauty salons, and plastic surgery clinics. The poor are left scrambling to capture at least a sliver of bodily capital, so valuable and yet so elusive.

What struck me about people like Amelia was their immanent critique of how unfair beauty standards were in Brazilian society. As soon as they began to talk about beauty, they began to remark on the unfair ways that they had been excluded from it—and their evaluation of this exclusion was an extension of a larger critique of other inequalities in Brazilian society. This awareness of beauty as a form of inequality contradicts the notion that plastic surgery patients are simply dupes of a patriarchal system that seeks to objectify women.[1] As Kathy Davis argues, plastic surgery can be understood by patients as a form of agency—a way to take control of their lives in a culture that has unfair beauty standards.[2] She, along with Victoria Pitts-Taylor and Virginia Blum, has warned against the tendency of feminist criticism to shame or pathologize plastic surgery patients for choices they have made within specific cultural constraints. Such criticism seems to portray the feminist critic as superior or more enlightened than the submissive, pliant patient.[3] Listening to the patients—taking their claims seriously—should not preclude a critique of the wider social forces they are enmeshed in and are grappling with, and about which they might have particular insights.

In an effort to privilege the stories of plastic surgery patients, I now turn to affect and focus on the everyday stories I was told by working-class

Brazilians about why beauty matters to them. As I argued in the introduction, I am less interested in the tiresome structure-agency debate—whether Brazilians' participation in beauty regimes is an aspect of coercion or self-determination (it can be simultaneously both)—and I explore instead how beauty circulates as a sign in Brazilian society. In other words, I see beauty neither as a straightforward form of oppression nor as an expressive act of liberation, because to reduce it to one or the other would be to miss how beauty produces an affective economy *between* bodies. Following Sara Ahmed's theoretical framework, beauty can be understood as an affective quality—a visceral sensation that cannot be located in individual subjects, but which accumulates in and sticks to subjects only as it moves between and through bodies, producing value.[4] Amelia's complaint that beauty was elusive for her, compared to the ease with which the wealthy acquired it, showcases the idea that beauty is a relational object—one is ugly only in relation to more beautiful others. As it accumulates on specific bodies and eludes others, beauty becomes a form of affective capital, generating an aesthetic hierarchy that defines who matters and who does not matter in Brazilian society.

Grosz, Clough, and Puar have alerted us to the fact that raced, classed, and gendered bodies cannot be reduced to identitarian political projects or to discursive formations—they are provisional assemblages, always in a state of becoming, but ones that nonetheless produce seemingly tangible surfaces.[5] Focusing first on class, then on gender, and ending with race, I explore how the beauty/ugliness dyad combines powerfully with other bodily signs and provides legitimacy to forms of inequality, simultaneously producing the terrain on which these forms of inequality could be questioned. I argue that beauty shows us how bodies assemble into coherent gendered, racialized, and classed entities within the Brazilian context. Beauty, in other words, is the key to understanding why the promise of belonging to the body politic is always conditional in Brazil, inevitably tied to one's appearance, and why some bodies are more highly valued in this affective economy than others.

THE PRECARITY OF CLASS

On most Sunday afternoons, Gilda and João's small home became noisy and joyful with the arrival of their children and grandchildren. As in most other working-class homes in the neighborhood of São Gonçalo, located an hour inland from the beaches of Rio de Janeiro, the patio served a social space where family and friends gathered. Gilda and João had been married for more than fifty years, and both were in their seventies and retired. On this particular Sunday, I was sitting on a wooden bench next to João and Gilda, looking through some family pictures. I saw a photograph of a woman who, in comparison, looked older than Gilda in the picture, and I asked whether this was Gilda's mother or an older relative. Gilda explained this was a picture of a deceased family friend who was Gilda's age, but who had gone through many difficulties throughout her life, including a laborious and unhappy job, a troubled marriage, and the death of one of her children. These had aged her well beyond her years, leaving her *acabada* (finished, spent).

I must have looked puzzled, because Gilda asked me to compare the appearance of her two elder grandsons, Carlos and Emilio, both of them in their thirties. Gilda pointed out that while Carlos had an office job and had clear, light skin from working all day inside a building, Emilio was a manual laborer who spent a large part of the day under the sun and thus had aged, burnt skin. João chimed in and began a long diatribe about how hard physical work was, and how much he had suffered as a railroad worker and a salt miner. The railroad soot, which had killed many of his coworkers, had damaged his lungs, too, and the mine salt had affected his eyesight and dried out the skin of his hands, now rough and calloused. Carlos and I should be very thankful, he said, for having an education and thus being able to avoid physical work. Gilda agreed, and added, "É o serviço que acaba com a gente" (It's our job that finishes us off).

From this exchange, one gathers that Gilda and João, like many other working-class Brazilians I interviewed, understand aging as an index of how hard a person's life has been. A person who is finished or spent is one whose appearance betrays a difficult past, registering on his or her body those indelible marks left by emotional hardships such as a troubled marriage or years of grueling work. The body testifies, in other words, about a person's struggles as a member of the working class, as well as the privileges afforded to those who can live more carefree lives. Gilda's contrast between her two grandsons, Carlos and Emilio, was a comment not only on their appearance but also on Carlos's upward mobility and Emilio's relative nonmobility. As the only one of her grandchildren who had attended college, Carlos had landed a white-collar job in a multinational company, which provided him with certain economic stability and benefits such as health insurance and guaranteed vacation time. Carlos was committed to his family and supplemented both his parents' and grandparents' limited incomes with his own, but he now lived a life that was nearly unrecognizable to Gilda and João.

At the time, I was rooming with Carlos in Copacabana, which afforded us immediate access to the beautiful beaches of Rio de Janeiro, its best-known touristic landmarks, and its thriving nightlife. His grandparents, however, very rarely ventured far from São Gonçalo and considered Copacabana to be too expensive and somewhat foreign. I was an element of that foreignness: an anthropologist who sometimes frequented their home on Sundays as a close friend of Carlos, but someone who was still out of place and whose life had been radically different from theirs, marked by high levels of education and geographic mobility. My body was different too—they remarked on how soft my hands were in comparison to João's calloused and hardened hands.

The body is a landscape on which memories are indelibly written because these past experiences become embodied sensorial events. As Nadia Seremetakis argues, the senses act as "record-keepers of material existence," conveying the social meanings given to bodily histories. The senses are a social medium of communication that, like language, provide meaning to embodied experiences, yet operate in a different register from language.[6] For instance, when João was reminiscing about his difficult work at the salt mines, he passed the index finger of his right hand over the palm of his left hand, as if tracing the past through the texture of his skin. Class is thus marked on the body in particular ways.

Carlos admired his grandfather's build and toughness from all those years of hard work, but it was not something he desired for himself. In fact, Carlos put a lot of effort and time into marking his own body as distinct as possible from the blue-collar bodies he had grown up around. Without fail, he went to the beauty salon every two weeks to get a haircut and a manicure (not an uncommon practice for men in Rio de Janeiro) and was fastidious about keeping his fingernails clean. He spent a considerable amount of money at the dentist's to whiten his teeth, and at the podiatrist's to smooth out any calluses on his feet. He did not do all those things because he had unlimited amounts of disposable income—on the contrary, he worried constantly about his growing debt and the daily expenses of living in Copacabana. When I asked him why he invested so much in his appearance, he told me that a "businessman would never hold an expensive Montblanc pen with damaged fingernails," and thus he would also never hire a person with hands that seemed to belong to a factory worker. Carlos was not embarrassed by the place he had come from (he was proud to take me to São Gonçalo), but he claimed that any small detail would be analyzed during job interviews for good white-collar jobs, and one had to play the part to get hired and then promoted within a company like the one he worked for.

Carlos was hyperaware of the ways that bodily aesthetics were markers of class position and class mobility, but he was hardly an exception. The working-class patients I interviewed named employment as one of the main reasons they were pursuing plastic surgery. In the waiting rooms of publicly funded hospitals, I commonly heard expressions like: "Beauty opens doors" and "Only beautiful people are successful."

For example, Josilene, a forty-seven-year-old woman who had worked for several years at a state agency, but who had recently become unemployed, believed that a breast-reduction surgery at the Santa Casa de Misericórdia would improve her chances at landing a new job:

> People don't look at your clothes, they look at your body. Women run a risk [when getting surgery], but if it is successful, as in most cases, it's worth it. . . . Appearance is important to have credibility and, from there on, to gain trust. It doesn't matter if one is intelligent or one has a degree; immediately it is appearance that counts. Only after the exterior does the interior matter. . . . Brazil is a developing country, and women work at home and outside of the home, in risky areas, and this ages you. Everything contributes: a good diet, too. . . . Stress causes premature aging. A person who makes a small salary, who doesn't eat well, and has a bad marriage is going to feel ugly.

Josilene understood that the body could be a much stronger class marker than any clothes she could wear, and she tied having the right appearance to credibility and success. She believed that working-class women like her aged prematurely owing to their small salaries, their stress from dealing with everyday risks such as crime, and their double shift at home and at work. Even though the surgery would cost less at the Santa Casa than at a private clinic, Josilene still had difficulty paying for it, given that she was currently unemployed. She was optimistic about how her life would be after the surgery, however, and felt she owed the surgery to herself, stating, "A woman who loves herself takes care of herself." She recognized the surgery as a risk, but felt the risk was worth it in the end because it was potentially a life-changing investment.

The working class frames its own quest for beauty as a constant struggle against daily problems and the effect of labor on the body. Working-class patients nearly always described their surgeries as *plásticas reparadoras* (reconstructive plastic surgeries), even if their surgeries would be considered aesthetic from a medical point of view. Initially, I believed that patients defined their surgeries as reconstructive simply as a maneuver to get them approved by the public system, since doctors commonly do the same to get the Brazilian public health-care system to cover the costs of aesthetic surgery, as I explained in chapter 2. I was surprised to see, though, that even at the Santa Casa, where aesthetic surgery could be purchased for a lower price and did not need to be designated in any particular way, the patients would still identify their surgeries as reconstructive. The description of surgeries as reconstructive remained consistent even when I interviewed patients long after their surgeries were completed, making me realize that patients were invested in that particular definition.

Even though the categories *aesthetic* and *reconstructive* derive from a medical distinction, working-class patients have laid claim to *plástica reparadora* as a morally justifiable form of plastic surgery. The word *reparadora* is particularly resonant in Portuguese, because it is a derivative of the word *repair,* and it allowed working-class patients to argue that they were repairing their bodies rather than enhancing them. Giovanna, a forty-two-year-old seamstress who had previously had a tummy tuck at a teaching hospital, and who was now considering getting a breast lift, told me that repairing her body had become a necessity. She argued that the kind of beauty she saw on television and in magazines was "only for those who have money," while "women without the economic conditions to take care of themselves become depressed." Giovanna explained that she was able to afford her surgery only after saving up for nearly two years, even though her surgery was for health reasons, and she contrasted her own quest for beauty with the ease with which the rich could find well-being.

I was struck by the degree to which patients' perceptions about beauty were grounded on their economic worldview, their personal histories, and their embodied experiences. For instance, a seventy-one-year-old retired washerwoman named Leonora told me that she felt that all her years spent washing the clothes of her clients had destroyed her hands, and that what she most wanted now was to remove the dark spots from her hands, so that she would be able to rest them and fully enjoy her retirement. Her memory of years and years of labor made an affective association between aging and the landscape of her hands, generating a perception of beauty that was unique to her experience. In other words, perceptions of beauty latch onto bodily features laden with sensory memories, which then experientially emerge as topographical sites of consequence on the body.

Diva, a fifty-five-year-old woman who worked in a transportation company and who wanted to get treatment for the varicose veins on her legs, also expressed how much her aesthetic issue was tied to her daily routine:

> I feel ashamed, especially at the beach. My body is whole, but it feels muti-lated. People of low income like me do not have money for a gym, we have to work and carry heavy things. My legs make me uncomfortable. I'm afraid of even showing them to my husband. . . . It's a problem I did not have in my youth; but at work I had to carry heavy things, and my busy life never allowed me to lie down and extend my legs. I would arrive home from work and go directly to the kitchen. That is why my legs are like this today.

Diva's daily burden as both a laborer and a housewife manifested itself as a physical burden as well, which shamed her and gave her the sensa-tion of being mutilated—of being an abject, partial body. It is as if the progressive taxation suffered by her body accrued through sensorial memories and became associated with ugliness. In her mind, this experi-ence was inextricably associated with her lower income: those with higher incomes never had to do backbreaking physical labor and, as a result, never had to feel the way she did.

Working-class patients repeatedly contrasted their own experiences of beauty with the presumed experiences of the wealthy because they experienced beauty as a form of lack—as a value that is generously bestowed upon those with money, but which for them was a precarious, largely inaccessible form of capital. If we understand beauty as a sign that gives bodies value only in relation to other bodies, we comprehend why working-class patients are so anxious about their appearance in relation to the difficulties of the job market and the neoliberal economic structures they have to navigate. People increasingly seek out beautifica-tion practices in times of economic uncertainty because beauty is per-meated by the affects of precarity—the disquiet and apprehension of knowing that one's economic position is inherently insecure.

As Anne Allison has lucidly argued, precarity is not only a condition of economic uncertainty characteristic of the neoliberal times we live in, but a form of affect as well, typified by the sense of anxiety and the feel-ings of being unmoored and directionless that are tied to economic inse-curity.[7] Allison's analysis is applicable to Brazil, but for my interviewees the forms of affect tied to uncertainty are felt in a way that resembles becoming unmoored or alienated from one's own body: Diva's body was whole but felt mutilated, whereas Amelia felt like the undead, and both framed their aesthetic procedures as necessary repairs to make their position a little less precarious in relation to others. In Brazil, precarity is tied to particular structures of feeling regarding the body and its value.

Working-class patients, however, also critique the fact that beauty is not equally accessible to everyone. They emphasize their own struggle to access beauty, and they see plastic surgery as a necessary repair for their bodies, in comparison to the purely aesthetic surgeries done by the wealthy. This point is important because most of the literature about plastic surgery in Brazil has portrayed it as a practice that the working class adopts simply as a way to imitate the upper classes. For example, Mirian Goldenberg has argued that Rio de Janeiro's middle class "are also often the vanguard for behavior in Brazil, given that what they do is valued and imitated by other segments of the population. . . . [T]he body-capital displayed by this group is far and away the most imitated body by Brazilians."[8] Alexander Edmonds similarly claims, "Demand for plastic surgery—as a symbol of modern femininity—is perhaps stimulated in a context where cross-class mimesis occurs between social strata living in intimate contact."[9] Both Goldenberg and Edmonds rely on Pierre Bourdieu's conception of cultural capital as a set of bodily dispositions (including aesthetic taste) that belongs to the dominant classes, and that is imitated by lower classes looking for upward mobility.[10]

My notion of affective capital refuses the idea that classed perceptions of taste are themselves being transmitted, and I claim that forms of affect are transmitted instead. The signs that provide bodily value cannot be said to reside within a particular class or to belong to a group that others then seek to imitate. Affective capital only provides value to bodies as a consequence of its circulation—everyone experiences beauty as a field of social relations in which some bodies accumulate more value than others. This experience of beauty becomes imbricated with embodied forms of precarity and personal experiences of labor, which give rise to topographies of beauty that are class-specific, as well as specific to one's individual bodily history. Reducing practices of beautification to imitation evacuates the ways in which bodies are relational objects that come into being within an affective economy of beauty.

THE CONTAGIOUSNESS OF GENDER

I had known Carlos for nearly a year before he finally shared with me the story of his plastic surgery. We were walking along Copacabana's famous boardwalk on a particular summer evening, enjoying the warm breeze and the sound of the waves, when he hesitatingly turned to me and said he had something to tell me. A few years back, he confessed, he had had liposuction to get rid of fatty tissue on his chest, which he believed gave him the appearance of having feminine breasts. I was surprised about this revelation, because he had been well aware that I was doing research on beautification practices, and we had chatted at length about it. I asked him why he had not felt comfortable about sharing this with me before. Carlos answered that he hid this procedure from everyone, even his family and his closest friends. He had always been embarrassed about the shape of his chest, and had been bullied about it by other kids at school. He was so self-conscious he refused to take off his shirt even during the hottest days of summer. When he got his first real desk job, he immediately began to save up for plastic surgery. It was a considerable amount of money—"I could have made a down payment on a car instead," he mused—but Carlos believed it had been worth it.

The surgery was done under local anesthetic in the doctor's office, which meant he remained awake throughout the procedure, and he remembered in detail how painful it was when the doctor inserted the small cannulas in his chest and sucked out the fat. The invasiveness of the procedure made him angry and uneasy—"It was the most painful experience of my life, and the doctor dismissed my complaints." At the time, he still lived with his parents, but he did not tell them anything when he got home. He simply wore the compression garment the doctor had recommended and stoically wrapped his swollen, sore chest on his own after each shower. Eventually, the inflammation subsided, and even though the difference in his body was minimal, it gave Carlos the confidence to begin taking off his shirt in public.

As I mentioned earlier, Carlos was the first in his family to land a white-collar desk job, which became a symbol of his upward mobility in relation to others in his milieu. The fact that his first large purchase was plastic surgery is symptomatic of the ways that beautification is associated with incorporating forms of bodily value and, thus, making tangible one's success, as precarious as it may be. It is also significant that Carlos chose to masculinize a part of his body that he considered to be unseemly feminine, and that he was ashamed about telling anyone he had undergone plastic surgery. He frequently spoke with his cousins and peers about going to the gym or doing other kinds of physical exercise—such bodily practices are considered appropriate ways for men to transform their bodies and become more attractive. One of Carlos's cousins was pretty open with his male friends about his use of supplements and steroids to gain muscle and lose body fat more quickly, which some considered to be unwise but not shameful.[11] Plastic surgery, however, was clearly considered a feminine practice by most of my interviewees.

Women were a large majority of the patients in the private and publicly funded hospitals where I carried out my research, and when I approached men I had difficulty getting them to open up about the reasons they wanted surgery. Those who agreed to talk to me emphasized strongly that their surgery would correct a medical issue, and that plastic surgery had been recommended by a doctor. The most common complaint among working-class men was the same issue Carlos had with his chest—a condition known as gynecomastia, or hyperdeveloped mammary glands on a male. My interviewees described the procedure to correct this condition as a way to look more manly and normal, perhaps in an effort to portray it as a way to remasculinize their bodies, despite the usual association between plastic surgery and femininity. Another surgery that is recently gaining traction among men is a form of liposculpture that provides men "six-pack" abs, and is also clearly tied to traditional gender norms of male muscularity and strength (see fig. 7).

Women, on the other hand, were much more comfortable about sharing their reasons for surgery and normalized their procedures as valid and necessary techniques to beautify the female body. Many women mentioned that they had female friends and relatives who had already undergone plastic surgery, and who had recommended they go through with it as well. Mônica, a working-class woman in her forties who came to the Santa Casa for a low-price tummy tuck, told me that her sister-in-law and a female cousin had gotten breast implants here, and her neighbor had undergone a breast reduction, and that all three were happy with the results. Mônica was uncomfortable with the stretch marks on her abdomen after having three children (one of them by C-section), and she decided to improve her appearance, despite the fact that her husband was not bothered by her stretch marks. Even men with big bellies, she said, could easily find younger women, so men did not quite understand what women went through.

Wanda, who used to work as a maid, said her husband worried about her face-lift and considered it unnecessary, but her son did not care either way and she had the full support of her daughter. She described it as longtime dream of hers, which many of her female friends shared; and she did not fear surgery, because she had undergone a C-section and a tubal ligation when she was younger. She hoped a face-

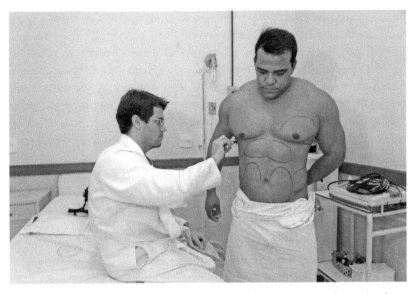

FIG 7. A medical resident marking the body of a working-class patient about to undergo a fat-reduction surgery to define his pectoral and abdominal muscles. Photo courtesy of Vincent Rosenblatt.

lift would provide her with new work opportunities, since she still had the strength and energy to iron clothes even in her sixties.

Nedite told me that when she turned forty she decided to make some improvements, which included putting on braces on her teeth and undergoing a breast lift to repair the effects of breast-feeding her two children. Her daughter and her female friends encouraged her, especially a friend who had undergone two plastic surgeries already. Nedite had been married for twenty years, and she thought it was silly that her husband cared so little about appearance and had let himself go, getting fat. Nedite believed that by valorizing her own body, she would make him less likely to cheat on her. She was aware that he surreptitiously checked out other women on occasion, even if he always denied it.

These women are unique individuals, but there are some clear commonalities threaded throughout their narratives, which reveal certain patterns regarding how gender intersects with beauty. First, many of these women felt that plastic surgery was a natural step following the surgeries they had had earlier in their lives, such as a C-section or a tubal ligation. These women, in Lawrence Cohen's term, were operable—they become interpellated as gendered citizens through their commitment to invasive surgical procedures, naturalized as inevitable aspects of a woman's life history.[12] Second, these women tied specifically feminine biological processes, such as giving birth and breast-feeding, to necessary repairs later in life, such as tummy tucks and breast lifts. Again, the language they used was *plásticas reparadoras*—their surgeries were a form of repair rather than a means of enhancement, but this time tied to their labor as mothers. Many of them understood plastic surgery as a form of self-care that represented the first time they would be cared for, as opposed to their caring for others.

Suely, a fifty-three-year-old maid from Belo Horizonte, described with pleasure the time that she spent in recovery after her tummy tuck. Even though it had been uncomfortable and painful, she recalled it fondly because her husband had taken care of her for a change. "I could not even bend over, so he had to wash my feet, . . . and I cried out for him to bring me food when I was hungry," she recounted with a smile on her face. She explained that cooking and cleaning would have been detrimental while she was healing after the surgery, and that her mother, daughter, and neighbors took turns caring for the household while she stayed in bed. Suely had obviously never before been able to relegate all responsibilities to others, which is why she found the situation remarkable. She added, "I did this to take care of myself after working a whole lifetime for others." Repairing the body, then, also represented a form of leisure and self-care that momentarily reversed the gendered relations of labor in Suely's life.

Perhaps the most important aspect of women's relationship to beauty, however, is the way that women share information about plastic surgeries with each other. Mônica, Wanda, and Nedite all expressed having learned about the possibility of plastic surgery from female friends or family members who had already undergone such procedures. They gained much more support and encouragement for their plans to undergo surgery from that female cohort than from the men in their lives, particularly their husbands, and were critical of men's ability to ignore beautification altogether. Compare this to the silence that surrounds men's plastic surgeries—Carlos underwent his in secrecy, unwilling to tell anybody in his life except his closest friends, and then only years after the event. There was little to no opportunity for Carlos's experience to become an example for others, and he never encouraged his male friends to get plastic surgery. Male interviewees, in general, saw such surgeries as exceptional measures to correct their misgendered bodies, while women portrayed them as routine ways to keep up the female body.

I am not simply arguing that women, more than men, pressure each other into surgery; my point is that by sharing personal histories and embodied sensations, women bring their bodies into operable subjectivity in ways that men do not. Beauty is a sign that circulates among women and assigns value to female bodies as an effect of that circulation, and medical practices of beautification are invested with affective significance because they seem to magically revalorize female bodies, reversing the effects of aging, procreation, and labor. Furthermore, women's bodies are portrayed as particularly vulnerable to aging in comparison to men's bodies: "Men age but women decay" is a popular saying I heard several times from interviewees. Women fully participate in the circulation of beauty as a feminine value; but men are reluctant to promote the idea of beauty as a masculine value, because they believe that it could render their masculinity fragile, and that they are meant to cultivate it in other ways, such as weightlifting. As a form of affective capital, in other words, beauty produces a contagious form of gender difference, in which women are more operable than men and women's desire for surgery is naturalized in ways that men's desire is not.

The literature on medicalization in Brazil has remarked on the astoundingly high rates of C-section, tubal ligation, episiotomy, hormonal therapy, and plastic surgery in Brazil, but most of it argues that these technologies are emblems of modernity that provide status and, therefore, are desirable to Brazilian women.[13] The argument becomes somewhat tautological at points: women desire modern medical technologies because the status of modernity is desirable to women. This emphasis on modernity as a causal mechanism does not explain why plastic surgery—which is not a gender-specific intervention—is highly desirable to women but much less desirable to men. As Rey Chow has argued, following René Girard, desire is the outcome of social relations, because something becomes desirable only when we notice that others also desire it. Desiring what others desire "is the primary event that engenders its own momentum and power of contagion. . . . Desire (like consciousness) is thus mimetic, to be located in the interstices of interactions between people."[14] I emphasize the ways in which women share their surgical experiences with each other in order to bring forward the insight that desire for beautification is first and foremost a contagious social relation, permeated by affect. Women listen to other women they trust, with whom they share strong bonds of friendship or kinship, before they ever set foot in a plastic surgery clinic.

Of course, gendered relations of power, and particular gendered histories of medicalization, thoroughly shape the circulation of gendered affect. While men like Carlos regarded plastic surgery as an invasive practice and were more ambivalent about the painful recovery it entailed, women had no qualms about submitting their bodies to surgical transformation. Two weeks after undergoing a breast lift, Nedite said that pain was a normal and bearable experience given the long-term benefits of plastic surgery, and that she looked forward to having other surgeries. Wanda told me that she was "willing to do anything that employed a scalpel" at the Santa Casa, because she had witnessed how well surgeries turned out under Pitanguy's purview. Gender mediated one's interpretation of surgical pain and one's trust in one's surgical future.

Nonetheless, it is important to consider the ways in which crossing the threshold of the clinic immediately subjected patients to a medical gaze highly invested in gender difference. While plastic surgeons see it as their duty to offer surgery to low-income individuals (for self-interested reasons as well, as noted in the preceding chapter), they do not believe everyone deserves such surgeries. Publicly funded hospitals have a series of requirements that serve as barriers to "problem patients." The two most important requirements are a physical examination and a psychological evaluation, which determine whether a patient's desire for surgery is medically justified and whether he or she is psychologically prepared for it. I attended several psychological evaluations and immediately noticed a difference between how male and female patients were assessed.

For example, the female psychologist at the Santa Casa was suspicious of a middle-aged man who wanted a face-lift, and who openly worried about aging, using language similar to that of female patients who desired the same surgery. The psychologist told me after he left the room that this patient was probably a homosexual, too concerned with his appearance, and thus a bad candidate for surgery. In contrast, surgeons and psychologists were highly sympathetic with male patients who complained about gynecomastia, and stressed to me how much that condition made patients suffer. One surgeon told me that gynecomastia "makes men feel their manhood is threatened," and that they are frequently called *mariquinhas* (sissies) by their male peers. Men's desire for a normative body justifies their surgery because it distinguishes their desire from simple vanity. Women, however, are encouraged to cultivate self-esteem through their bodily appearance, and surgeons rationalize that Brazilian women suffer particularly intense social pressure to conform to beauty standards, in a way that men do not. It is a surgeon's duty to relieve that psychological suffering and provide women with better self-esteem by transforming their bodies.

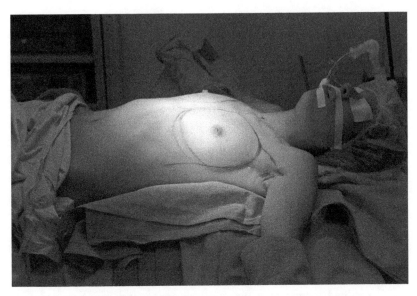

FIG 8. A working-class female patient about to undergo a breast augmentation surgery. Photo courtesy of Vincent Rosenblatt.

Surgeons never examine, however, how their own discourse constructs women's bodies as always lacking or in excess of the norm. Not only were women's surgeries more likely to be approved by the medical staff at publicly funded hospitals, but also women's bodies were subject to a much wider range of diagnoses than men's bodies. Gynecomastia was one of the few surgeries specifically designed for male bodies, along with rare cases of penile enhancement and testicular implants (for men who had been born without testicles or who had lost them in an accident or through disease). Women's breasts, abdominal area, buttocks, thighs, and sexual organs, on the other hand, were all subject to a few different types of diagnoses, each requiring a different treatment. Breasts, for example, could be enlarged, reduced, lifted, or repaired—and the list of medical conditions imposed on them seemed almost endless, making the breast a central focus of surgical intervention (see fig. 8).

On one occasion, a mother brought her teenage daughter to the Santa Casa because they believed her breasts were abnormally small, and they were relieved when the doctor concurred and offered a specific diagnosis for the girl's condition: "hypotrophy of the mammary glands." Naming the condition not only justified silicone implants for the teenager but also supplied medical confirmation that the girl's body was indeed abnormal and in need of treatment. Similarly, a woman in her twenties who went to a federal hospital complaining of having an atypical vagina, which made her uncomfortable when wearing a bikini, was approved for a "nymphoplasty," or the surgical reduction of the vaginal labia. The surgeon who agreed to the surgery explained to me that large vaginal labia could sometimes produce abnormal sexual behavior, such as lesbianism or nymphomania, and thus the surgical correction was not merely aesthetic but also had a clear medical indication. This moralizing medical discourse served to reaffirm the notion that plastic surgery is a thoroughly heteronormative science, which produces more masculine men and more feminine women while simultaneously curtailing nonnormative genders and sexualities.

Given doctors' penchant for reinforcing the gender binary, it is not surprising that gender-variant individuals are the ones who have the hardest time getting access to plastic surgery in Brazil. In 2008, the Brazilian public health-care system began covering sex reassignment surgery for transgender patients. However, only four hospitals in the whole country are accredited for carrying out these surgeries, and they have stringent requirements for patients. Patients have to undergo two full years of counseling and prove to a psychiatric team that they indeed have gender identity disorder—a problematic diagnosis on its own.[15] Additionally, the medical emphasis on genital surgery as the defining element of what constitutes true transsexuality excludes from medical care many individuals, particularly those who identify as *travesti*. According to Don Kulick's and Marcos Benedetti's ethnographic accounts, *travestis* are the most common gender-variant subjectivity in Brazil, and even though they transform their own bodies through female hormones and silicone injections to gain feminine forms, they usually have no desire to alter their sexual organs.[16]

Travestis have to resort to self-transformation because they are routinely denied access to feminizing surgeries, such as breast augmentation, in publicly funded hospitals.[17] When I asked the lead psychiatrist at one of the four accredited hospitals why they refused medical care to *travestis*, he answered, "*Travestis* have no intention of removing their sexual organ, and they are more theatrical; while transsexuals are different because they are more discreet and want to be women sexually." He delegitimized the identity of *travestis* because they did not fit his idea of transsexuality or his classed expectation that women are discreet and demure. As I have argued elsewhere, this stringent definition of transsexuality, which defines the sexual organ itself as the locus of indisputable femininity, renders the gender identity of *travestis* as medically illegible and thus makes them ineligible for surgery.[18]

At the publicly funded hospitals where plastic surgery is offered to the general population, *travestis* are routinely turned away, something I witnessed firsthand. A *travesti* called Carol came into the Santa Casa one morning, her boyfriend in tow, and she waited patiently in the queue for a shot at a medical evaluation. Her expressed desire for breast implants was similar to that of other women, who were approved for the surgery, but Carol was open about her gender-variant identity. Shortly thereafter, she was denied the breast implant surgery she desired, and she left angrily, shouting she could not be denied a right given to everyone else. In the days that followed, the story of her denial circulated not only among the medical staff at the Santa Casa but also among doctors in the other hospitals I frequented—and a mocking, disrespectful tone was always employed to describe her desire for surgery. I highlight this story not only to showcase the discrimination Carol suffered but also to underline how much beauty mattered to her as a form of becoming.

As Julieta Vartabedian has argued, "Beauty enables *travestis* to be legible, to disclose their feminine shapes and the efforts made to achieve them. . . . [B]eauty—in its continuous doing—is what gives sense to their everyday reality and existence."[19] *Travestis* go to great lengths to become beautiful, and they are highly admired in Brazilian society for their ability to achieve feminine beauty, despite the widespread discrimination they face.[20] Several normatively gendered women I interviewed expressed awe at the beauty of some *travestis* and hoped they could achieve similar results through surgery—*travestis* seemed to confirm the very malleability of gender. In other words, notwithstanding the medical attempts to curtail expressions of beauty and reinforce the gender binary, doctors do not have a full monopoly on what beauty means in Brazil. Plastic surgeons attempt to reinscribe a very limited view of what is beautiful, and as gatekeepers of the medical system they determine which bodies get access to key techniques of beautification. Beauty, however, has a contagious affective value that has been disseminated beyond the confines of medical discourse. In the field of social relations, beauty circulates in unpredictable ways that allow for different forms of becoming, some gender normative, and some less so.

THE VISCOSITY OF RACE

Carlos is lighter-skinned than most people in his neighborhood in São Gonçalo. As in other working-class neighborhoods in the state of Rio de Janeiro, almost everyone there works in factory jobs or in low-paying service jobs, and a large majority of the population is visibly of non-white descent. Carlos's father and uncle, for example, are a much darker hue than he, which Carlos attributes to their being from the state of Bahia, widely considered to be the most African state in Brazil. Carlos looks more like his mother, who is mostly of Portuguese descent and is light-skinned, but he has his father's hair and nose and identifies as *pardo,* or racially mixed.

Carlos began to notice the privileges granted because of his light skin early on. When he got his first job as a teenager, working for a pizza chain in his neighborhood, he was surprised by the deference with which other employees of the same rank treated him. He later discovered that his coworkers had assumed Carlos's light skin (in contrast to theirs) must have meant he was a relative of the pizzeria's owner, who was light-skinned as well, and they expected he would get promoted to manager soon. After he got promoted in record time, he wondered how much his appearance was a factor; his boss had taken a liking to him very quickly and trusted him more than his other employees. With the money from that job, Carlos was able to go to night school and get a business degree at a local college. His grades were average, but with the degree in hand he began to apply for desk jobs in established businesses and landed one in an important multinational company. It was an entry-level position, but it paid more and had better benefits than any job his father had ever had. The pizzeria owner was sad to see him go, but was happy for his professional advancement—he had sometimes treated Carlos like a son.

At his new job, Carlos soon realized that he was not quite white enough. The multinational company he now worked for was located not in São Gonçalo but in the much wealthier neighborhood of Niterói. Carlos was proud of the job he held in the firm's accounting branch, but he described himself and those ranked at the same level as peons, doing the everyday grunt work, and he noticed many of them were from working-class neighborhoods. Except for the directorship of the company, held by foreigners, most of the managerial positions were assumed by white Brazilians—white in a way that Carlos was not—who had grown up in upper- or middle-class neighborhoods where people tend to be lighter skinned.

The one time that Carlos let his Afro-textured hair grow more than a couple of inches, he was criticized by a superior for having an unkempt appearance and told to go to a barbershop more often. From then on, Carlos kept his hair cut so short that it was impossible to tell its true texture. Women who were ranked in the same position as him, Carlos found out, all straightened their hair religiously, for similar reasons. His only dark-skinned work colleague, who also kept his hair short, complained that despite several decades of loyalty and competence he had been denied a promotion to a managerial position time and again. Carlos was skeptical that racism was behind this reluctance to promote his black colleague, until he, too, began to be passed over for promotions. He was particularly angry that a blonde, blue-eyed man who was younger than him and had much less experience was put directly in a managerial position and treated more leniently when he made serious mistakes. Carlos concluded that this young man either had someone higher up in the company vouching for him, or his *boa aparência* (good appearance) was behind his success in the company. Carlos was sometimes wistful about his time spent as a manager in the pizzeria, even though he made less money back then, because he had felt more valued.

Anthropologist Kia Caldwell observes that the racialized history of the phrase *boa aparência* is not neutral. When it became illegal in 1951 to state an outright preference for white applicants in job advertisements, *boa aparência* became a common euphemism for whiteness.[21] In 1995, the phrase *boa aparência* was banned as well, but the affective weight given to having the right appearance for any jobs associated with upward mobility remains an unstated truth that Brazilians know they need to navigate. The phrase does not simply apply to skin color— it is a polysemic concept that includes physical attributes like hair and teeth but also perceptions of hygiene and fashion, and it is highly contextual. For example, Carlos's experience demonstrates that he had the right appearance for a managerial job in the service industry in his neighborhood, and for an entry-level white-collar job, but perhaps not the appearance necessary for a management job in a company.

As a form of discrimination, *boa aparência* is powerful precisely because it is so diffuse and hard to corroborate—one can never be sure if appearance was indeed the cause of a perceived advantage or injustice, or whether there were more obscure forces at play, such as familial connections. Carlos was uncertain whether the pizzeria owner treated him like a son because they shared physical characteristics the other employees lacked, or whether he simply liked his personality; ultimately the reasons for this affinity might have been unconscious. Sometimes, however, *boa aparência* becomes more explicitly about race, like in the case of a job consultant who described good appearance as "always within a more common prototype: slim, light skinned, with *traços finos* [fine features]. People look not only for beautiful individuals, but for a standard type of beauty that is not exotic or different."[22] Again, context is key to interpreting this claim, since it would seem spurious to say that light skin and fine features (as opposed to nonwhite features that are commonly described as "flat" or "wide") are standard elements of beauty in Brazil—until one realizes that the job consultant is referring to middle- and upper-class forms of employment, where dark-skinned individuals would indeed be exotic fare.

The polysemic meanings of *boa aparência* are key to understanding the ways in which beauty becomes a racializing affect, generating value for certain features like lighter skin, blue eyes, straight hair, and a thin nose, while rendering all other features undesirable and unsuitable for those who hold well-paying jobs. Race itself comes into being only as an aggregate of these contingent forms of value given to physical features; and given the variety of phenotypes found in Brazil, race produces a wide range of bodily values that do not necessarily cohere into concrete ethnicities or racial identities.

The literature on race in Brazil has long described the country's color classification system as fluid, ambiguous and multiple,[23] because color is a highly contextual and situational category. In Brazil, color is a continuum rather than a set of fixed categories, and it is interpreted according to individual characteristics, not according to familial descent. This emphasis on fluidity contrasts, however, with ethnographies that describe the persistent, intimate forms of racism experienced by darker-skinned Brazilians, particularly in connection to the aesthetic devaluation of blackness in the public sphere.[24] Many scholars have struggled to reconcile the seemingly pervasive forms of racism in Brazil with the inconsistent or invisible patterns in which these forms of racism latch onto particular bodies. By focusing on beauty and *boa aparência*, I want to point out that phenotypes are valued or devalued only as an effect of how these racialized signs circulate between and through bodies—race or color does not exist independently of this movement tied so intimately to aesthetic evaluation. Therefore, racialized bodies materialize at specific junctures where forms of affective value accumulate in relation to some physical characteristics but not others, and this effect does not always correspond to concrete ethnic identities or to consistent forms of discrimination.

Jasbir Puar and Arun Saldanha have theorized that race has a viscous quality to it, sticking to certain body parts, to forms of clothing tied to religious practice, and to assemblages of bodies in messy ways, yet race is nonetheless contingent, localized, and tied to larger processes in the body politic.[25] I was surprised, for example, to find that physical characteristics I had never before perceived as tied to race were described as deeply racialized by my interviewees. For example, I met Julia, a woman in her sixties, at a federal hospital in Rio de Janeiro when she accompanied her ten-year-old grandson, who was getting ear surgery. She explained that this surgery was key to his future success:

> He needs to fix his ears so he won't have the same problems as his mother and father. . . . His mother and father made him wrong; he came with a manufacturing error, so now he needs fixing. . . . People have plastic surgery done so they are not different from others; to feel included in their social group; to not have those ears, that nose, those lips that cause suffering. . . . *Boa aparência* is important to be successful in the job market; people who say that is not the case are just saying that outwardly but think differently. Only in a *concurso público* [exam-based public position] they will have to hire you if you are smart, even if you are black. For all other professions, though, appearance is important, very much so. The talk about everyone having the same opportunities is just demagoguery.

In Julia's evaluation, *boa aparência* is a form of value that is elusive yet impossible to ignore. Investing in her grandson's surgery so early meant investing in a whole lifetime of opportunities that could otherwise be denied to him. Julia believed his protruding ears were a "manufacturing error"—an inheritable family trait—that had already caused problems and suffering for his parents, as markers of difference. The ears had become racialized like other characteristics that Julia associated with blackness, such as noses and lips. Despite her and her grandson's relatively light skin, Julia made explicit how the official discourse of racial equality is simply demagoguery. Without the surgery, her grandson would be in the same precarious position as black job candidates, who are consistently discriminated against.

There was a specific temporality to surgery associated with correcting racialized characteristics, particularly noses or ears. Unlike the surgery more closely associated with repairing the marks of motherhood or of heavy labor on the body, which was meant to reverse the effects of time, the correction of protruding ears or wide noses was frequently done early in life. As Julia did with her grandson, it was common for adults to bring their children in for surgeries that they perceived as preventive, and which they always described as necessary for their child's personal and professional realization as an adult.

For example, Ana Paula brought in her fifteen-year-old daughter, Marilene, to a teaching hospital for a nose surgery, which she said "had nothing to do with vanity." They had moved to Rio de Janeiro from the northeastern state of Ceará ten years earlier, and since then Ana Paula had noticed how much *preconceito* (discrimination) people showed against northeasterners and against those who were dark-skinned or black. Marilene was teased frequently at her school for being different, and she asked for the surgery as a way to fit in. Ana Paula had to take a break from work to help her daughter with the surgery, and it was a significant expense for her and her husband, but they both agreed it would help their daughter a lot in the future. Ana Paula stressed how one's appearance was crucial not only in the job market but also in any relationship one had, by improving conviviality with others. "Only the rich," Ana Paula said, "can easily make themselves beautiful, even if they exaggerate at times and end up with noses that are too thin and unnatural." For Ana Paula and her husband, there was a clear hope that a nose surgery would create a future for their daughter unlike the one reserved for them as northeastern migrants. Surgery promised to shelter Marilene from the racialization that had been imposed on the whole family and that had seemed to attach to their bodies; it was impossible to shake off unless a portion of Marilene's body became surgically disassociated from its origins.

Leila, a fifty-five-year-old social worker who was slightly dark-skinned like Ana Paula and her daughter, but who had experienced a more comfortable life owing to her father's stable career in the military, described how much her nose surgery had meant to her when she turned eighteen. She had been shy, unsure of herself until then, and the surgery helped her gain the self-confidence she had today. Her father found a way to get her the surgery in a military hospital, and her mother helped her during the recovery period. "It really helped with my self-esteem," she told me. "I felt very ugly due to my wide nose, because the nose is the center of everything. *Aparência* [appearance] is so important, for one's job, for one's romantic life, and for one's personal life. Unfortunately, people value appearance so much, and there is discrimination. I believe Brazilian women are vain because there are so many beaches, and the body is freely exposed. There is so much sensuality in Brazil due to the black and Indian heritage." Even though Leila connected her nose surgery to the discrimination she could potentially face, she still valued the sensuality of the body she explicitly tied to blackness and indigenousness. She seemed to make a distinction between what was considered beautiful for one's body and for one's face.

Leila made that distinction for her children as well. She said that one of her daughters, Marisol, was happily married to a German man, whom she described as being attracted to her daughter's uniquely Brazilian qualities: "She is affectionate, she is bronzed, and she takes care of her body." What made Marisol's face beautiful, however, was a "harmonious nose," which Leila compared to the nose of the white supermodel Gisele Bündchen. Her other daughter, Tânia, had unfortunately inherited Leila's ugly nose, and she had sought to correct it through surgery after separating from her husband, even though it was very difficult financially. Leila fully supported her daughter's nose surgery, which she felt provided "a harmonious, subtle result—no one notices she had surgery—and it brought her happiness." She was less supportive, however, of bodily surgeries like silicone implants and liposuction, which she felt were signs of excessive vanity. Leila said one could get those bodily shapes naturally, simply by dieting, and that nose surgery was different because it provided real opportunities in life.

For some interviewees, like Leila, racial difference was not an explicit reason for surgery, but it clearly lurked beneath, an unspoken source of unease, tied to the importance of *aparência* in society. Leila clearly valued the nose of her daughter Marisol more highly because it was a whiter nose that reminded her of Gisele Bündchen's German heritage, while her own nose and the nose of her daughter Tânia were imagined as distant from that "harmonious" ideal before surgery. She also felt plastic surgery could help with her daughter's difficult situation after her separation, and thus surgery was about creating a different future. The "black and Indian heritage" Leila described, however, seemed relegated to the past, an erotic legacy that created sensual bodies for all Brazilian women.

I return to this important notion of harmony and its relation to whiteness in chapter 5, but will point out here that the materiality and viscosity of race make it particularly hard to shake off or simply wish away. The racialization of features haunts the body and forecloses some possibilities for happiness while opening others, but it is always perceived as having a real, very tangible effect on how one relates to others in Brazil. The phrase *boa aparência* was by far the most common reason my working-class interviewees gave for why beauty matters in Brazil. Even if the surgery they were getting seemed to be related more to the wear and tear of physical labor or attributable to their gendered labor as mothers, *boa aparência* was a constant refrain that indicated a pervasive concern with the lurking presence of racial discrimination in their lives.

THE PLEASURES AND TYRANNIES OF BEAUTY

Beauty is a complex form of affective value that, in its circulation, produces gendered, raced, and classed bodies. Each of those bodily properties are experienced, at a visceral level, in different ways within Brazil's aesthetic hierarchies. I threaded the example of Carlos throughout the chapter, however, to illustrate that any one individual experiences these sometimes contradictory forms of becoming simultaneously, not separately. Carlos's concern about how his appearance might influence his precarious upward mobility intersected with both his desire for a more normatively gendered body and his experiences of racial privilege and racial discrimination. Beauty was important to him because it condensed the race, gender, and class hierarchies he had to navigate every day. He and many others described beauty as a tyrannical and yet pleasurable force in their lives. Beauty was something they could not risk living without, because ugliness meant different forms of social exclusion. But beauty was also something they relished, that they felt would provide them with happiness, and which they desired intensely for themselves.

Let me return for a brief moment to the São Gonçalo home of Carlos's grandparents, Gilda and João, which I enjoyed visiting during the big family gatherings they hosted on Sunday afternoons. Gilda and her three sisters were full of a vitality that I have rarely seen in a group of women of any age, much less among women in their sixties and seventies. They always teased and bantered when I dropped by, and we played a little game that said much about the affective significance of beauty. They asked me to decide which one of them was the most beautiful that day, then burst into laughter at my shy responses and thought of reasons why I had made the wrong choice. The purpose was not only to poke fun at an anthropologist of dubious sexuality but also to playfully claim beauty for themselves in a society that said they could no longer be beautiful and worthy of recognition. Then they would tell me stories of how they had once been the most beautiful sisters in the neighborhood, and how many men had wooed them. As they reminisced about their escapades during long-gone Carnivals, they would begin to sing well-known Carnival tunes and dance to them.

Our little game about beauty allowed them to collapse the past into the present and replay embodied histories of pleasure. Focusing the ethnographic lens on actors who desire and value beauty allows us to become attuned to the affective dimensions of beauty and recognize that beauty matters precisely because it is a form of becoming that cannot be reduced to the agency/structure dichotomy. Rather than understanding beauty as a force imposed on subjects or a form of empowerment emerging from within them, beauty is a relational object that happens only between subjects, in that game of recognition we play with each other.

CHAPTER 4

Hope, Affect, Mobility

In one of Rio de Janeiro's most famous favelas, Cidade de Deus (City of God), teenage girls walked up and down a makeshift catwalk in the community's small basketball court for their biweekly lesson in the local modeling school called Lente dos Sonhos, or Dream Lens. I observed them from the bleachers while sitting next to the girls' mothers and other curious passersby who had gathered to look at the girls and cheer them on. Their teacher, a young model from the community called Giovanna, gave the girls tips on how to sway their hips as they walked on high heels. She demonstrated how to pose twice at the end of the catwalk and look ahead at imaginary cameras taking their pictures, before twirling around and walking back. Some girls looked nervous and self-conscious, obviously uncomfortable about being the center of attention, while others carried themselves with confidence and a contained excitement, taking the class very seriously and professionally.

I asked one of the mothers sitting next to me why she had enrolled her daughter in a modeling class, and she answered that many people had commented on her daughter's beauty and encouraged her to try out for modeling. "Who knows," she said with a gleam of hope in her eyes, "she might get lucky and get discovered. Then she can make a career out of this and guarantee her future." The modeling school allowed the girls to practice becoming a model and thus produce the beauty their mothers hoped would become a real source of income in the future. In Portuguese, the verb *se produzir* (to produce oneself) is used to describe the process of embellishment through makeup, hairdo, clothing, and physical performance. Mothers described their daughters as becoming *produzidas* (produced, beautified) when they accomplished beauty through labor on and through the body. Thus, beauty is seen not as an inherent quality of the body but as a transient, affective quality that can be practiced, learned, and improved.

There was hopeful anticipation in every step these girls rehearsed, because it meant incorporating a gendered performance associated with success and upward mobility. The hope that beauty can take a girl out of poverty resonates powerfully in Brazilian society. Narratives of upward mobility through beauty are interwoven throughout diverse forms of media—from journalistic accounts of recently discovered models, to the carefully crafted storylines of soap operas and beauty pageants. The media's fascination with the million-dollar contracts for Brazilian models who strut the catwalks in Milan, Paris, or New York produces these women as admired icons of a valuable femininity that is exported from Brazil to the whole world. Models who come from poor backgrounds are frequently portrayed in the media as "Cinderellas" touched by a magic wand, transported from poverty to the idealized world of fashion.[1]

As the name Dream Lens suggests, it is only through the lens of a camera that a girl's unrealized potential is thought to blossom into tangible economic success. I found out about Dream Lens because there was a flurry of media coverage congratulating the school for its initiative and its ability to, as one newspaper stated it, "transform poor girls into models," and for putting "fashion at the service of [promoting] citizenship."[2] One article showed a picture of Giovanna, the favela's most successful model and instructor, posing in front of the Eiffel Tower in a fashionable jacket, skinny jeans, boots, and long, straight hair, as proof of this veritable "carioca fairy tale." The photograph was meant to symbolize the wonder of "social inclusion" through beauty, which brought the "daughter of a maid and a fruit seller" to Paris for the "career of her dreams."[3] Ironically, it was only after Giovanna was seen as having transcended her origins—by performing the mobility, cosmopolitanism, and success associated with transnational fashion—that her beauty was understood as having become a valuable asset for herself, her community, and the nation as a whole.

During the class, Giovanna rarely boasted about her accomplishments, but she always carried herself as a model would, having mastered all the small details that made her presentation on the catwalk convincing. When Giovanna walked flawlessly down the runway, the improvised catwalk made of old rugs held down with bricks began to fade away, yielding the spotlight to the powerful model taking the stage—her head high and her body focused on the prize. Through her perfectly tailored gestures, Giovanna communicated a sophisticated femininity that symbolized a more luxurious world than the one her students knew and experienced every day. Learning to perform beauty as Giovanna did was a way to access that world, even if only for a fleeting moment.

This almost magical transformation held despite the fact that Giovanna had in reality found it difficult to book many modeling jobs, had gone to Paris only once, and found that her material conditions barely changed after she began modeling. She still lived in her humble one-room home in City of God and dreamed of one day parading the catwalks of famous designers in Europe. The magic of make-believe is not simply an imitation exercise; it is an affective attachment that promises girls from poor communities that they can transcend their reality via the outside recognition of their beauty. The founder of Dream Lens, a local photographer called Mauro, acknowledged that very few, if any, of the girls who take the modeling course would actually make a living from modeling. For him, though, teaching the girls to value their own beauty was a source of motivation and self-esteem—for themselves and for the community as a whole. Learning how to "take care of themselves" would lead to job opportunities in areas where appearance is fundamental, like the beauty industry and receptionist jobs. He told me he believed the modeling school "rescued these girls from prostitution or from becoming pregnant at a very young age," because it gave them something to look forward to. In this way, beauty was seen to fundamentally change their lives.

Beauty is understood not simply as an attribute to be imitated but as a quality imbued with what Sara Ahmed calls the "promise of happiness"—in other words, it prompts the anticipation of a better, more fulfilling life. Furthermore, this promise of a better future becomes a moral injunction insofar as it links happiness with good, virtuous behaviors.[4] Mauro, for example, believed not only that beauty would lead to better economic opportunities for the young girls he photographed, but also that it would preserve these girls' sexuality from the dangers of sex work and unwed motherhood. The sexuality of women from favelas, and of Brazilian women of color in general, is frequently coded as excessive and in need of intervention.[5] The narratives that link beauty to upward mobility, therefore, also construct an idealized image of the poor young women who deserve this mobility, sexualizing and racializing them in very particular ways. Before I delve into these narratives, however, I develop a bit further the idea that beauty becomes a form of economic value in society, and I discuss what that says about beauty as a form of labor.

THE VALUE OF BEAUTY

Affective labor has garnered renewed theoretical attention recently, particularly after Michael Hardt and Antonio Negri's claim that this type of labor, along with intellectual labor, is becoming hegemonic in post-Fordist capitalism, replacing the primacy previously held by industrial labor. Affective and intellectual labor, they argue, are immaterial forms of production that generate emotions, relationships, and subjectivities, collapsing the divide between private and public spheres and rendering labor more precarious and flexible. Affective labor is largely feminized, evidenced by the predominance of women in the service economy and in jobs where affect is central to labor performance, as is the case with nurses and executive assistants.[6]

Hardt and Negri acknowledge their indebtedness to the Marxist-feminist literature that first recognized the importance of women's affective work within and outside the family, but they do not pursue gender as an analytic to understand precisely how affect produces subjectivities, or why it has become predominant today. The consequence, as Leopoldina Fortunati points out, is that Hardt and Negri's work, like that of other Marxist authors, reduces women to their bodies and naturalizes their association with emotional work.[7] I would add that their reliance on a transcendent category like the "multitude" is a gesture that, in subsuming gender and race under class difference, does not fully account for the ways in which different forms of inequality intersect with one another. Hardt and Negri's insights point, nonetheless, to an important shift in the global modes of production within society—from forms of labor that produce goods and services alienated from the worker's body, to forms of labor that produce affect by embodying production itself and establishing work as a form of self-making. The commodity or service to be sold is now incorporated into the worker's own subjectivity, possibly producing new forms of alienation from one's very self, but also producing novel forms of resistance.

If affective labor has indeed become a hegemonic form of social organization, we should analyze how it deploys gender difference to generate value and produce subjectivity. The 1970s Marxist-feminist debate on women's labor initially asked the question of whether the unpaid labor of women at home, where they care for the needs of the whole family, is central to the social reproduction of capitalism. Scholars argued that femininity itself was a product of the private/public divide that was necessary to capitalism, constructing a realm of the personal where women were said to naturally belong and where their labor alleviated the alienation of male laborers.[8] Kathi Weeks argues that in the effort to map domestic labor onto the needs of Marxist production, Marxist-feminists had a tendency to value housework over other affective forms of care that are less tangible; this reified the distinctions between the domestic and the public spheres.[9]

The insight that affect could be considered a productive and active form of work, however, led Arlie Hochschild, among others, to argue that feminized pink-collar jobs (such as the work of flight attendants) also require workers to perform emotional labor, managing the emotions of clients through their own performance of feminine care for their well-being. Not only is gender productive, in the way it performs a familiar code of femininity and maternalism associated with domesticity, but also gender itself is produced through this type of labor, having deeply constitutive effects on the subjectivities of workers, including the men who choose to work in those jobs.[10] Taking seriously Hardt and Negri's claim that post-Fordist capitalism collapses the divide that exists between private and public life, one could argue that affective labor spills beyond the domestic realm into all areas of social life, bringing along the constitutive effects of gender associated with this new mode of production.

I argue that the definition of affective labor should not be limited to the types of labor that require caring for others but should be extended to any type of labor that produces gendered affects rather than tangible commodities. Performances of beauty can be understood as a form of affective labor, where the product itself is not separable from the act of production. Beauty is a practice of self-making as well as a form of work, one that crafts the producer's subjectivity at the same time that it generates value on and through the body. I consider beauty, in particular, to be a gendered form of work that produces the body itself as valuable, especially when the labor of beauty is performed in relation to an imagined audience that will evaluate and visually consume the body in question as a commodity.

Elizabeth Wissinger has argued that models do not manage the emotions of clients directly, but become conduits for affective energies that interpellate viewers both consciously and below the level of awareness, attracting attention to the images and products marketers want to sell.[11]

Modeling requires the constant upkeep of the body and the collapse of the intimate life of the model into his or her public life, because the model's own body becomes the product that is constantly assessed and measured by the fashion industry.[12] Additionally, the images of models never reach the consumer in an unmediated manner, but are carefully manipulated and managed by a whole team of industry experts who embed particular narratives in photographic shoots and runway shows.

It is through this process of mediation that affective labor transforms into capital. In the previous chapter I defined beauty as a form of affective capital that provides bodies value through the circulation of classed, racialized, and gendered signs that accumulate on some bodies but not others. Affective capital has a distinct use-value and exchange-value for the subject who excels at forms of beauty work and whose body evinces the signs of attractiveness—my interviewees insisted that beauty not only improved their sense of self-worth but also improved their bodily worth in relation to others and provided real economic opportunities. The advantages provided by beauty, however, cannot usually be quantified in economic terms with any exactitude, because affective capital is an ineffable, indistinct, and precarious quality.

It is only in professions like modeling and in beauty pageants—where beauty becomes alienated from the individuals who embody that quality, and it is packaged, sold, and exchanged as a commodity—that beauty transforms into a tangible form of economic value. Beauty becomes a capital-producing commodity, in other words, only when it produces surplus value for others besides the model or beauty queen within the commodity chain, particularly the industry experts who discovered those beautiful subjects in the first place. In Brazil, public culture celebrates not only the beauty of models and celebrities but also those who discover them—reaffirming the gendered Cinderella narrative of beauty leading to recognition by an assumed male viewer, who then magically brings these women out of poverty. Mass-mediated texts fetishize the process of discovering beauty, rather than valuing the congealed labor-time that went into producing it. Performances of beauty seem to acquire economic value only after they are recognized as beautiful by diverse forms of media, and after the mediatized representations of this beauty begin to circulate within the public sphere as commoditized cultural texts. The affective labor of beauty thus congeals into alienable forms of capital.

It is a particular form of affect, hope, that mediates the gap between performances of beauty that have utility for an individual, and performances of beauty that become fetishized as idealized, commoditized narratives of becoming within public culture. This hopeful form of affect interpellates viewers who consume such captivating rags-to-riches narratives, rejoicing in the unexpected transformation of elusive affective capital into tangible economic success. If beauty is so laden with hope, it is because there are limited possibilities for upward mobility in Brazil. There are almost no guarantees of equal access to housing, education, or employment,[13] producing a precarious future for most low-income households. As Ghassan Hage argues, one of the basic characteristics of capitalist society has been its capacity to produce the hope of achieving upward mobility in all individuals, even in the face of massive inequalities. As post-Fordist capitalism renders such hope more fragile, by undermining the role of the state as guarantor of the population's general welfare, individuals take to magical means that still produce hopefulness in the face of uncertainty.[14] Jean and John Comaroff have similarly pointed out the global rise of occult economies that aim to magically produce value out of nothing, in the context of the widespread insecurity produced by late capitalism.[15]

In Brazilian society, beauty is intrinsically associated with the promise of happiness because the human body is both the site from which added value directly emanates and the site where it accumulates, and everyone possesses a human body, no matter how far removed one is from power, wealth, or connections. The magical value of beauty seems to be within reach in ways that other forms of mobility are not. Additionally, contemporary capitalism's magic thrives on forms of aesthetic pleasure, as Nigel Thrift points out, because it is a force that produces shared capacities for gratification.[16] Nowadays, immaterial forms of labor and value seem more real than obscure forms of capital accumulation that are inaccessible to most of the population, and they shimmer particularly brightly in the narratives crafted for our television screens.

THE ICONICITY OF WHITENESS

I was sitting next to Marcella in her São Gonçalo home one Saturday evening, watching *Viver a Vida* (Seize the Day), the nightly prime-time soap opera, when she mentioned how ugly the baby on the screen was. "What an ugly child!" she exclaimed. "How unfortunate for her mother, although she is to blame for it, too." Marcella disapproved of this particular character in the soap opera, a middle-class black woman called Sandra, who had had opportunities to marry up but chose instead to marry a poor black man living in a dangerous favela. Every other character in the soap opera, black or white, disapproved of this union as well, and constructed it as a moral failure on Sandra's part. It eventually resulted in Sandra's downward mobility and put at risk her own safety and the health of her baby. Marcella, however, also disapproved of the baby's appearance, a blackness that she thought could have been avoided if Sandra had married someone who was lighter-skinned. When I pressed Marcella further, she contrasted it to a real-life situation, a niece of hers who, despite being *morena,* had married a blue-eyed young man who owned a shoe shop nearby. "She made the right choice and was able to *melhorar a raça* [improve the race]—her children are so beautiful!"

I was surprised by Marcella's analysis, since her sister had married a black man from Bahia, and she had never said anything remotely racist before then. As Elizabeth Hordge-Freeman argues, however, women in Brazil are frequently judged for the aesthetic qualities of the children they produce.[17] Marcella interpreted Sandra's failures, therefore, as reflected in the ugliness of Sandra's baby. In the context of the soap opera narrative, Sandra was clearly the foolish sister, in contrast to her beautiful sister Helena, who demonstrated more wisdom by marrying a wealthy white man. Helena's main conflict, as a heroine, consisted in succeeding as a supermodel and in finding acceptance within her husband's family, following the typical storyline in soap operas, where a woman's beauty leads to upward mobility and success. Helena's other struggle was her difficulty with having children, which led to her divorce, but the last scene of the soap opera shows her second white husband happily holding their first child, a very light-skinned baby who represents Helena's success as a mother and a woman. According to Jasmine Mitchell, it is through reproduction that blackness is domesticated in telenovelas, particularly when it is tied to the whitening of the nation.[18]

Marcella was rooting for Helena, but she was a minority compared to other television viewers. The actress who played Helena, Taís Araújo, is one of the most highly recognized black actresses in Brazil, and she was making history at the time by playing the first black female lead in a prime-time soap opera. Owing to the high level of audience rejection, however, the writers of *Viver a Vida* shifted the storyline based on feedback they received from polls and discussion groups. They began to develop the story of another supermodel—Helena's white rival, Luciana—who winds up quadriplegic after an accident, and who struggles with feeling beautiful and finding love as a disabled individual. The character captured the imagination of the audience in a way that Helena did not. Even today, Taís Araújo's character is one of the prime-time heroines with the greatest level of rejection by Brazilian audiences,[19] and it seems unlikely that Brazilian television will repeat the experiment of having a black female lead anytime soon.

Traditionally, Brazilian soap operas cast black actors only in stereotypical roles such as chauffeurs, cooks, maids, mammies, and in other subaltern positions in relation to the main, lighter-skinned characters.[20] More recently, black actors have portrayed corrupt politicians, wily social climbers, and seductresses. Taís Araújo's portrayal of Helena, however, followed a role reserved for white female leads: that of the *mocinha* (good girl, maiden) whose virtue and honesty hold up in the face of a series of obstacles that prevent her from finding happiness, success, and true love. The unpopularity of Brazil's first black *mocinha* demonstrates that women whose beauty is worthy of such recognition and mobility are inevitably coded as white and must follow a racial script as well as a gendered script to fulfill their potential.

Ethnographic accounts of television, like Purnima Mankekar's and Lila Abu-Lughod's analyses of serialized dramas in India and Egypt, have pointed out the ways in which these cultural texts create archetypical images of womanhood, nationhood, and modernity. These hegemonic narratives about women's lives, however, are not passively consumed by target audiences, but are actively interpreted in relation to the daily concerns of viewers.[21] The pleasures of spectatorship, in other words, do not depend on audience members agreeing or disagreeing with the hegemonic narratives presented in these serialized dramas. As Anne Allison argues, the affective appeal of new entertainment media, and their potential to generate economic value, relies instead on their capacity to generate new modes of information-sharing, attachment, and sociality.[22] More recently, Mankekar has argued that affect is particularly useful in understanding public cultures, because it explains how mass-mediated texts engage audiences at a visceral, sensuous level. Certain iconic images—such as women's bodies—become indexical for larger notions of heterosexuality, tradition, sensuality, and family and generate specific forms of affect that circulate between and across subjects. Affect thus "blurs the boundaries between private feelings and public sentiments" producing "webs of relationality" that transcend the individual.[23] In Brazil, women's bodies have a similar iconicity within mass-mediated texts, but always in relation to their perceived beauty.

Brazilian soap operas are cultural texts of utmost importance within the national context. In the most powerful television network in Brazil, Globo, they make up a large part of daily programming and employ some of the most talented writers, actors, and art directors in the country, incurring up to $250,000 in production costs per episode.[24] These high production values are more than justified by the profits garnered nationally through advertising, as well as by the resale of transmission rights to networks from more than 130 different countries in the international market.[25] As a genre, the Brazilian soap opera is considered an accessible form of leisure for all Brazilians that is capable of influencing public discussion about sensitive topics, like family, love, intimacy, social injustice, and politics.

As Esther Hamburger argues, soap operas are so important in the Brazilian public sphere because they represent national concerns in the form of family dramas, blurring the distinction between the public and the private, and the intimate and the political, as well as between the fiction and nonfiction genres. The spectator uses the national lexicon provided by soap opera narratives in order to discern who deserves success in the national sphere.[26] Not only Marcella, but also other people I watched soap operas with, made moral judgments about characters from soap operas, deciding whether to root for their success or wish for their downfall. These characters represent archetypes from Brazilian society that are gendered, classed, and racialized in particular ways. For example, the sudden reversal of social positions, which places the poor above the rich and powerful, is a common plot device in soap operas that provides comic relief, yet it is always temporary and never redemptive, unlike the *mocinha*'s narrative of enduring upward mobility through beauty.

For the *mocinha*, the plot generally takes one of two routes: she is either from humble origins and must confront the villains who prevent her from succeeding, or she is initially wealthy and loses everything to conniving villains, from whom she must then strive to recover what is rightfully hers. The *mocinha* is usually portrayed by some of the most beautiful and talented white actresses in Brazil, and the beauty of the actress becomes a central linchpin of the character's path out of poverty and into love and success. The *mocinha*'s beauty is equated with upward mobility because it is what provides her a new job opportunity, like a modeling career, or what makes her attractive to a wealthy *galã* (male lead). The white male lead is very much a Prince Charming who sweeps the *mocinha* off her feet and offers her a better life, going against social conventions.

The villain is usually characterized as someone who disapproves of this union and will do anything to stop it, or as a female competitor who envies the *mocinha* and wants the male lead for herself. At least a couple of soap operas (*Mulheres de Areia* [Secrets of Sand], aired in 1993, and *Paraíso Tropical* [Tropical Paradise], aired in 2007) featured twin sisters with opposite personalities: the good twin, who is genuinely in love with the wealthy male lead, and the evil twin, a gold digger who wants to take her sister's place by manipulating her way up the social ladder. Even though in both soap operas the same actress played the parts of the *mocinha* and the villain, it was relatively easy to tell them apart on screen, because the evil twin wore heavier makeup and dressed more sensuously than her sexually modest good twin. Given that these plots relied frequently on one sister impersonating the other, however, it was up to the scriptwriters and the actress to give the audience subtle clues about who was the "real" sister under the costume.

Soap opera performances are carefully managed to communicate different affects depending on the character's personality and provoke specific reactions in the audience. Actors who play villains in a given soap opera usually complain that fans approach them on the street to berate them for their character's wrongdoings—such is the emotional attachment that the audience develops for particular narratives. When the *mocinha* loses the sympathy of the television viewers, on the other hand, the ratings of a soap opera can quickly plummet. The virtuous femininity of the *mocinha* is a performance that serves as a moral compass for the narrative as a whole. Since the message crafted by soap operas is that female beauty is a double-edged sword—providing power and mobility to both good and bad women—the humble personality of the *mocinha* can never come into question as she pursues her dreams. Otherwise, she is likely to bear a resemblance to the overly ambitious villains. At the same time, she needs to show strength of character in order to confront the villains who are out to destroy her, thereby providing a redemptive narrative to the plot.

Female lead actresses walk a fine line in terms of how they play a role, therefore, while male leads do not suffer the same pressure. The reason for this difference is that masculine beauty is not portrayed as redemptive. Even the male heroes are portrayed as promiscuous and easily susceptible to sexual advances from female villains, without the need of romance. The beautiful and desirable *mocinha,* however, will have sexual relations only with her true love, and even if she falls for a villain's false vows of love, her love for him is genuine and pure. The upward mobility and happiness she achieves by the end of the soap opera (usually culminating in her wedding to her true love) are portrayed as a fair reward for her untarnished qualities.

This moral tale about femininity is meant to appeal to the middle-class and working-class women who are considered the core audience of soap operas. The iconicity of the *mocinha*'s performance allows the audience to respond affectively to this idealized Cinderella story, where beauty allows women of humble beginnings to transcend their origins. The hegemonic definition of beauty written into soap operas, however, demonstrates that not all types of beauty possess the affective value that can then translate into economic capital and upward mobility. The *mocinha* might be poor, but she is usually lighter-skinned or has lighter eyes than most the women of her social class. She is recognized as beautiful by the male lead because, despite having a menial job, she stands out as someone who physically does not appear to be working class.

The soap opera *Belissima* (So Beautiful), which aired between 2005 and 2006, made the recognition of white beauty a recurrent theme central to the plotline. In a flashback scene that was aired in the first episode and repeated several times throughout the duration of the soap opera, we saw the *mocinha* Vitória as a poor white girl living on the streets, selling candy at a stoplight to the drivers passing by, with her younger brother beside her. When the handsome, green-eyed Pedro looked out of the window of his expensive car, he was awestruck by her beauty; he offered to buy the whole box of candy Vitória was selling, which took her by surprise. Their dialogue was interrupted, however, when an unidentified man threatened to hit Vitória's younger brother, and Pedro stepped out of his car to defend the boy, saving them both. The camera then focused again on Vitória, zooming in beyond her torn clothes and dirty hands to display only her beautiful face, her light eyes hopeful and expectant as she looked back toward Pedro, who was now smiling at her. No dialogue was necessary to explain that this was the beginning of a Cinderella story, and that Pedro would marry Vitória despite the objections of his grandmother, the powerful businesswoman Bia Falcão.

Bia Falcão, played by the celebrated actress Fernanda Montenegro, was a fascinating character because she seemed to judge everyone according to their appearance. She doted on her great-granddaughter Sabina (Pedro and Vitoria's daughter), who was light-skinned and red-haired. She was particularly harsh to her granddaughter, Júlia, for not having the good looks of her dead mother, who was a model. She plotted to have the family fortune taken from Júlia by hiring a blue-eyed con man, André, who used his good looks to seduce Júlia, marry her, and then proceed to steal all she had. It was unclear why Bia Falcão hated the normatively beautiful Vitória, until the end of the soap opera, when we discover that Vitória is actually the illegitimate child of Bia Falcão, whom she abandoned at birth. In other words, Pedro unknowingly married his own aunt, having recognized in her the beauty of the upper class to which she rightly belonged all along. By rescuing a beautiful white woman from poverty, he was really rescuing one of his own. The soap opera thus constructs Vitória's whiteness as a symbol of her true social status, even though it never expresses this in words. Instead, whiteness becomes an iconic referent of hopeful forms of affect, reinforcing the association between the *mocinha*'s white femininity and upward mobility.

There was surprisingly little comment about the plot twist involving incest in the public reactions to the soap opera's final episode, or in any conversations I had about it with Brazilian viewers. People focused instead on how Bia Falcão escaped to Paris with an attractive male hustler—some were upset that she was not punished for her villainy. Other people focused on how a former villain in the soap opera, the con man André, was willing to jump in front of Vitória to save her from Bia Falcão's bullet. As he is dying, he confesses to Júlia that he always expected to get far in life owing to his good looks, and that he was sorry to have used them for nefarious means. The entire soap opera thus constructed beauty as a form of capital that provides mobility, but gendered it in different ways. Only a woman's beauty could become an untarnished source of mobility, if she remained honest and sexually pure, while a man's attractiveness always remained morally dubious.

SCOUTING FOR SAMENESS

The fairy-tale narrative of the young *mocinha* who is recognized through her beauty has found new life in beauty contests that seek to discover models. Several of these contests are held nationwide, including Menina Fantástica (Fantastic Girl), held by the Globo Network, Elite Model Look, held by a modeling agency, and Faces, held by a department store, to name only a few. Most of these contests have strict age limitations and are seeking to discover teenagers or very young adults. I focus here on a contest called "Beleza na Favela" (Beauty in the Favela), because it in particular reveals the hopeful forms of affect communicated by these beauty competitions.

"Beauty in the Favela" was a popular segment of the morning variety show *Hoje em Dia* on the Record Network from 2007 to 2016 and had several editions during that time. The premise of the contest was to send scouts to some of the poorest communities in Brazil looking for teenage girls who had the potential to become models, and then transport them "from the [urban] peripheries to the catwalk."[27] Each segment would begin in the favelas of a given Brazilian state, where the modeling scout would pick one among dozens of girls who had enthusiastically signed up to compete. The show would then shift to the television studio in São Paulo, where a panel of judges decided which girl would represent the state in the national finals. The move from the favela to São Paulo already signified a transcendent move to modernity, as represented by the flashiness of the television studio. It was also stressed that this was the first time the girls had boarded a plane and traveled so far from home, all for the "dream of being a model so they can help their families."[28] The contestants were very careful to stress that they were looking to help not themselves but their parents and their community, thus disavowing any ambitious tendencies that might be considered unseemly. These girls were represented as models of behavior for all other teenagers and not simply as models of beauty.

The scholarly literature on beauty pageants argues that such events build national communities by constructing femininity as a symbol of national unity, citizenship, and pluralism, even as they define respectable womanhood as sexually proper and racially unmarked.[29] I add that beauty contests also offer the hope of a better future for contestants and their families, because they are able to transform beauty into tangible economic value. In "Beauty in the Favela," these teenage girls' recognition as beautiful on national television was meant to symbolize a form of social justice that would include the Brazilian poor in the larger national community. As one television host put it:

> Winning "Beauty in the Favela" is not simply winning a beauty contest, it is defeating prejudice, defeating the difficulties and obstacles, defeating social difference, and showing to all Brazilians, all the population, that Brazil is much more . . . than the neighborhoods of the South Zone of Rio de Janeiro and the South Zone of São Paulo, those that we see on television every day. Brazil is a country that has in its most impoverished communities great values, great talents that only need to be discovered. That is the Midas touch of our program, through the reporters who went forth and made their discoveries.[30]

The stated purpose of "Beauty in the Favela," then, is to conquer prejudice and social difference by revealing unknown beauties obscured by the poverty of their surroundings. One presenter compared it to "revealing the diamond hidden in the favelas of Brazil."[31]

This discovery of an unrecognized Brazilian natural resource, as it were, positions the television program as a progressive and nationalistic enterprise. The accomplishment of transforming these girls into models is portrayed as uplifting their entire communities, by reinstating these forgotten Brazilian peripheries into the national imaginary through the beauty of their young women. Beauty is represented as a valuable product that can be consumed within Brazil or exported abroad, aligning these girls' hopes with hopes of national progress. By positioning itself as the facilitator of these discoveries, the program becomes an arbiter of what is beautiful and who deserves to be hopeful. This authority is enacted through the self-congratulatory "Midas touch" of its scouts, who are commended for venturing into uncharted territory.

What was worthy beauty in the eyes of these scouts? First of all, the teenage girls who were chosen were tall and thin, since the ability to compete within global modeling standards was a prerequisite. As I followed the program, however, I also noticed that the scouts almost always looked for the girl who seemed out of place because she had lighter eyes while the rest had brown eyes, or because her nose was thin and pointy while the others had larger noses. Long, straight hair was not a precondition but seemed a very desirable quality. The girls who were chosen might be dark-skinned, but not exaggeratedly so. The scouts looked for a type of beauty that might be uncommon in the communities they visited, but which is ever-present in Brazilian television and advertising, including among the scouts themselves. The scouts did not verbalize their criteria, however; they just presented their choices as the natural recognition of a beauty that beckoned to them. In short, the scouts looked for girls who would be considered beautiful in the wealthy South Zone of Rio de Janeiro or São Paulo, the same aesthetic the show criticized as being ubiquitous on television.

The scouts never bothered to ask what the people in the communities they visited might admire as beautiful, reinforcing the idea that the periphery can be revalued only by acquiescing to the standards emanating from the metropolitan centers. The panel of judges that decided who would be the finalist from each Brazilian state reinforced this choice, weeding out racial difference and, perhaps unconsciously, making the contestants as uniform as possible. Brazilian beauty is thus constructed as homogeneously single, a whiteness that might be tinged with a hint of racial mixture but not overwhelmed by it, similar to the beauty norms that Marcia Ochoa describes as "miss-ing race" in Venezuelan pageants.[32] I watched the show with my friend Priscila, a young black woman in her thirties, and without my prompting her, she agreed that the show had a suspicious slant toward whiteness. "Why don't they choose more girls with my hair type?" she complained. A writer for the leftist magazine Caros Amigos agreed, accusing "Beauty in the Favela" of "reinforcing the beauty hierarchy of whiteness promoted by the media since the very first soap operas."[33]

Contests like "Beauty in the Favela" claim to promote *inclusão social* (social inclusion), a term widely used in Brazil to describe any number of governmental and nongovernmental programs that attempt to redress social inequality. In the context of beauty pageants, however, the term functions as an affective anchor that reassures television viewers that beauty indeed produces upward mobility for the poor, while simultaneously reinforcing the aesthetic judgments that exclude a majority of the Brazilian population from the citizenship made available by beauty. The winner of "Beauty in the Favela" in 2008 was Vanessa, a very light-skinned girl from the northern state of Amapá, whose population self-identifies as 75 percent brown or black, according to the latest government census.[34] She was not necessarily the most eye-catching of all the contestants, but she was the most confident on the runway and seemed to have the most previous experience. In a biographical sketch about Vanessa aired the next day, the program stressed not her appearance but rather the work that she had put into becoming a model. Members of her family had taught her how to walk and behave like a model when she was very young, and she had remained faithful to that dream. The victory was merely the beginning in Vanessa's journey, one television host stated, since now she had to learn how to navigate the complex modeling world in order to succeed.

As Rebecca King-O'Riain argues, the work necessary to naturalize a certain physical appearance as beautiful within a community is an accomplishment—the product of a "bodily, cultural and political effort to assert, maintain and challenge" the meanings of racialized and gendered performances.[35] Beauty contestants should not be seen as passive actors who are simply identified as beautiful. On the contrary, they actively participate in shaping and embodying their own subjectivities in relation to the expectations of what models should be like, requiring extensive affective labor on their part. Beauty contests craft a given version of femininity as a form of economic and social capital, which contestants and their parents can consciously appropriate and deploy. Despite being from humble backgrounds, several of the finalists claimed that modeling had been their objective since childhood, demonstrating the long-term investment in transforming a girl's beauty into capital.

In a 2015 journalism piece aired on Globo's program *Profissão Reporter* (Profession: Reporter), girls who dream about becoming models were portrayed as selfless heroines sacrificing everything for their families, and as vessels in whom families invest their hopes for economic advancement.[36] A fifteen-year-old teenager, Josy Carvalho, was featured as the new discovery of Dilson Stein, the same modeling scout who had discovered Brazil's biggest supermodel, Gisele Bündchen. Josy was very light-skinned, had light eyes and long, straight hair, and was tall for her age. Her humble family had taken out loans worth thousands of dollars to enroll her in modeling schools and to produce her modeling portfolio, which showcases professional photographs of Josy. At the time of the journalistic piece, however, the investments had not yet paid off—the hopes invested in her potential were on hold until she got older and started booking jobs. Josy was clearly emotionally invested in this career as a way to provide for her family, and she cried for the camera as she described the car and nicer home she would purchase for them once she began making money.

The economic capital produced by beauty remained speculative for Josy but had clearly paid off for the modeling scout, Dilson Stein, who described in the news piece how he, too, had come from poverty, before showcasing his huge home. Based in Horizontina, Rio Grande do Sul, he never needed to go far from home to discover the models that made him wealthy, because, as he explained, 40 percent of all Brazilian models come from that particular state, despite the fact that it possesses less than 6 percent of the total Brazilian population.[37] The piece does not explain the reason for this disparity but simply assumes that the viewer is aware that Rio Grande do Sul's advantage lies in its history of having had a higher proportion of white European immigrants than other states. Josy Carvalho was recognized as beautiful because she fit this European standard of beauty and lived in a city neighboring Horizontina, close to Stein's scouting eye.

As I explained in chapter 1, the construction of a Brazilian geography of beauty harkens back to the early twentieth century and imagines the southern regions of the country as possessing more beautiful men and women because they have higher proportions of European heritage. The models who became famous and confirmed Dilson Stein's scouting prowess are all very light-skinned, have features associated with Europeans, such as small noses and straight hair, and have European-sounding last names: Bündchen, Ambrosio, Tentrini, Linzmeyer, Sulzbach.[38] In the Globo network's modeling contest, "Fantastic Girl" (a segment of the Sunday variety show *Fantástico*), a modeling scout made explicit why fashion models are discovered in southern Brazil more than in other regions: "Like [in] any other location in Brazil, one finds centers of miscegenation, and in the South the concentration of Italian, German, Polish and other ethnicities is particularly strong, which then mix with the Brazilian and reveal many beauties every year. . . . Talking about genetics, the [southern girl] has a strong link to the European features desired in the international market, but we cannot discount that Brazilian beauty found in other Brazilian states is also successful here and abroad."[39]

We see here how the logic of miscegenation portrays Brazilian beauty as a mainly European inheritance that becomes slightly nationalized through mixture, yet still retains the desirable European features that translate into a valuable appearance. The scout makes it clear that beauty can be found in other states as well, but it is portrayed as much rarer—a scout would clearly have less trouble finding beauty in the southern regions of Brazil than elsewhere. It is common for modeling agencies and beauty contests to blame the preference for European features on the international market; but the claim is spurious, because there are many darker-skinned Brazilian models, like Laís Ribeiro, who are more successful abroad than in Brazil. Whiteness, however, is understood as a form of cosmopolitan capital in Brazil, a quality that gestures toward a universal, unmarked beauty that scouts recognize as an economic form of value. Families like Josy's are encouraged to invest not only their time and money in this form of bodily capital but also their hopes of upward mobility.

Modeling and talent agencies traffic in hopeful forms of affect because managing these potential celebrities is a very profitable business, no matter how many of their clients make it as models or actors. Agencies charge high fees and commissions to help parents book auditions and casting calls for their children and to guide parents through the process. They also offer courses to improve the children's acting and modeling skills and to teach them how to behave during an audition. Every agency critiques the others for profiting from parents' high expectations while claiming that they truly have these families' welfare in mind. As evidence of their rate of success, their websites show examples of children and teenagers who started at the agency and are now famous models, soap opera actors, or advertising stars. The people who run these agencies, however, admit that very few of the children represented by the agency will actually book important jobs and make a profit, and even fewer will make a living as actors or models when they are adults. Nevertheless, the agencies never reject a candidate altogether, recommending instead that the child or teenager take more courses, lose some weight, or get braces to improve his or her chances.

When I asked the director of an agency in Rio de Janeiro why only white beauty seems to be valued in the industry, he answered that there was nothing they could do to include more diversity in mainstream media and advertising—it went against the very logic of selling a product. He explained, "If [the models] have the appearance of coming from an upper social class it works out; if they have a bad appearance, like teeth with cavities, the product will not sell. . . . Many advertisers demand [that their models] have light eyes and light hair because it represents high class." Beauty, therefore, is a form of value that affectively revalues other commodities with which it becomes associated, but only insofar as it provides the whiter appearance of the Brazilian high class. The surplus value that can be extracted from beauty to create capital, in other words, is a highly racialized and classed form of value, limiting the chances of success for the majority of children and teenagers enrolled in these agencies.

Parents of all racial backgrounds remain hopeful, however, despite all odds. I interviewed several working-class parents at one of these agencies in Rio de Janeiro, all of whom expressed with emotion the bright future they envisioned for their child. A mother who lived in Rio's working-class North Zone commented how difficult it was to find a normal job in Brazil, even with an education. She hoped her nine-year-old son could instead become an actor, since he had shone during casting calls and nearly got the part for a film. Beauty was relative, she explained to me, because "some people have light eyes but they still lack any charm," unlike her son. Everyone in the family encouraged her to continue investing in this agency after seeing how well the professional pictures of her son came out.

Neide, who worked as a bank teller, recounted how much coming to this agency was driven by the wishes of her thirteen-year-old daughter:

> People would approach us in the street and say that she could be a model. She was always attracted to fashion and used to playfully imagine she was walking down a runway at home. I waited, however, until she asked me for this herself. It's important that I do this for her, and if it works, her fulfillment will also be mine. . . . My nephews also come to this agency, and began sooner than my daughter because their mother used to participate in beauty pageants, and they all have blue eyes and blond hair, so they had the initiative. Until a short time ago they only selected blue-eyed children for modeling, but now I see several types of beauty in the business. I believe my daughter has the beauty of a model and has the style for it.

I was struck by the fact that these two mothers were aware of the value of white features like light eyes and blonde hair in the acting and modeling industry yet maintained a fierce conviction that their children would still succeed. They asserted that whiteness was not the only form of capital that was valuable, and that there were more intangible characteristics, like "charm" or "style," that could trump the inherent value of whiteness. It was confirmed by the public recognition given to these children by friends, family, and even strangers on the street. Nonetheless, there seemed to be an inevitable advantage for people like Neide's nephews and their mother, who, owing to their physical features were almost expected to have the "initiative" to look for this type of profession.

In the bodies of children, as representatives of the future, beauty represents "the promise of happiness" in a different way than it does in adults.[40] Every possibility seems laid out for them, and parents relish this potentiality, unwilling to foreclose any possible futures for their children. Many parents I talked to insisted that they were not favoring acting and modeling over getting an education, and said they also invested in their children's sporting potential, such as soccer or gymnastics. Beauty, however, seemed to promise an especially glamorous future, one characterized by celebrity and superstardom.

Adelaide, a black woman who worked as a maid, imagined a fantastic future for her five-year-old child:

> I find my daughter to be so beautiful and decided to bring her to the agency. I bring her because she enjoys it; if she didn't, we would leave. I would love for her to become famous and to become a great actress like Taís Araújo or Beyoncé, who are such beautiful black women. Maybe she will one day work with Will Smith! We already went to a casting call, but it didn't work out. Because I pay for it, no one objects about the talent agency, not even her father. . . . People in this room find her beautiful, and this is a place already full of beautiful children.

Adelaide was proud of her daughter's blackness, styling her daughter's natural hair rather than straightening it (Adelaide's own hair was straightened), and favorably compared her to black celebrities. She did not permit anyone to criticize the hope she put in her daughter's beauty, not even the girl's father, and seemed optimistic that what is defined as beautiful would not be the same for the next generation—putting her daughter on par with the whiter "beautiful children" in the room. Not every parent, however, felt their children were valuable as they were at present. A military captain explained that he brought the daughter everyone recognized as beautiful because she was tall and thin, and that her younger sister was "a little chubby" and thus did not have a future in the agency unless she lost some weight. He hoped that his older daughter, only ten years old, would become a future beauty icon, but he was aware that the chances were slim.

Such hopefulness could perhaps be described as an instance of what Lauren Berlant calls "cruel optimism"—an attachment to political modalities that undermine the very well-being of the subjects who hold them dear, who cling to them nevertheless because they provide continuity to "the subject's sense of what it means to keep on living on and to look forward to being in the world."[41] Beauty constantly beckons to a future just beyond one's grasp, and is so seductive because it gives meaning to the belief that a better future is possible. This hope relies on the deeply held conviction that if Brazil is not yet a color-blind racial democracy, it ideally should be one, a dream that Robin Sheriff argues cuts across social classes.[42] It is also intimately tied, according to Donna Goldstein, to the nationalistic celebration of Brazil's supposedly color-blind erotic democracy, which masks the racial and sexual logic that underpins interracial desire.[43]

If television programs celebrate the mobility of young maidens, and if modeling and talent agencies for children and teenagers are able to draw in so many committed parents, it is because these forms of recognition seem more innocent and disguise the sexualized power relations that structure Brazilian inequality. The figure of the maiden or the child—innocent and desexualized—seems to sanitize the recognition of beauty as an egalitarian gesture. As Lee Edelman claims, the figure of the child also pushes us to invest in a political vision that is always a vision of futurity rather than one of the present.[44] The affective labor that goes into youthful beauty places the realization of one's hope for upward mobility in the future, seeming to always require additional labor to become a reality—and making it easier for agencies to alienate that labor for profit. Parents already see the value of their children's beauty; but in order to transform this value into capital, they require the recognition of modeling scouts and the media. This promise of recognition can be perpetually delayed, permitting scouts and the media to traffic in the hopes of parents and their children without ever fulfilling the dream of truly expanding the hegemonic definition of beauty.

SHORT-CIRCUITING HOPE

If there is an overdetermined, repetitive aspect to the hope devoted to beauty, it is because affects sometimes animate social circuits that seem hardwired, retracing the same trajectories time and again, as Kathleen

Stewart argues.[45] This does not mean, however, that beauty is inevitably tethered to those familiar circuits—like electricity, the intensities tied to beauty can shock and pleasure in unfamiliar ways, short-circuiting the narratives of upward mobility that tie beauty to hope.

Since 2003, the central market in Rio de Janeiro, known as the Saara, has promoted a yearly beauty contest to elect a Garota da Laje, or Concrete-Roof Girl. The *laje* is the simple flat roof made of concrete that is typical of working-class homes in Brazil, which, unlike a finished roof with tiles, allows the homeowner to add another level to the structure if necessary. This common practice of slowly building and adding to one's own home, which anthropologist James Holston calls "autoconstruction," allows working-class families to continuously personalize their homes according to need and lay claim to membership within their community through homeownership.[46] The architectural aesthetic of autoconstruction is considered ugly by upper- and middle-class Brazilians because, by displaying the concrete and bricks that constitute the house's structure, it refuses the appearance of being a finished product that one could purchase. The *laje* is a particularly important element in the architecture of an autoconstructed home, because it also serves as a space of socialization during hot summer days. Given that in Rio de Janeiro most working-class neighborhoods are located far away from the beach, it has become customary among working-class women to suntan themselves on the concrete roofs of their homes. The Concrete-Roof Girl contest not only recognizes this gendered beauty practice but also contributes value to the type of working-class housing that gives rise to it. The organizer of the beauty contest portrayed the aim of the event as "transforming the corny into a craze, [and] showing the beauty of the *comunidade* [favela, community] and the periphery."[47] The Concrete-Roof Girl is thus a representative of feminine beauty and of an architectural aesthetic valued by the working class.

The contestants of the Concrete-Roof Girl contest are not expected to be perfectly beautiful or highly *produzidas* (produced, beautified). The contestants are not very tall, thin, or young, and are of every hue available in Brazil. Many of them are already married and have children. As a contestant explained, the only requirement for contestants is "to have natural beauty, because no one here has had cosmetic treatments or plastic surgery, everybody has cellulite, everyone is natural."[48] The visible, natural imperfections on the bodies of these women are, like the noticeable construction materials in their autoconstructed homes, held up as evidence of authenticity. The contest thus provides a space for women to express their discontent with the idea that beauty cannot be a personalized aesthetic, but should be a mass-produced, uniform product of labor.

Another contestant, who worked every day at a bakery shop, exclaimed, "Brazil needs to find its true identity. . . . The Brazilian woman is *mestiça* [racially mixed], she needs to wake up at 4 am to work, and does not have the time to go to a beauty salon."[49] By emphasizing the racial diversity and busy working schedule of the average Brazilian woman, this contestant points out the fact that hegemonic representations and practices of beauty are largely inaccessible to them. The Concrete-Roof Girl contest celebrates beauty but does not seek to create a narrative of upward mobility associated with beauty. The prizes are not large amounts of money or fancy modeling contracts but, rather, a seven-year-old car (the winning prize), a plastic pool, a premolded *laje*, a barbeque grill, a stereo, and R$199 (about one hundred dollars) to spend at R$1.99 stores at the Saara market.[50] These are prizes associated with nonconspicuous consumption and with leisure, like the weekend barbeques that take place at the *laje*. Hopes for immediate and communal enjoyment replace the hopes for future success.

The contest garners plenty of media attention owing to its uniqueness. Much of the coverage is tongue-in-cheek, joking, for example, that "in the land of the *Garota de Ipanema* [Girl from Ipanema], the Concrete-Roof Girl has reached new heights."[51] Another reporter, pointing to a black contestant, argued that here indeed was the real "body of the Brazilian woman, full of curves, full of thighs. You don't have to be a [supermodel like] Gisele Bündchen. . . . [Y]ou can eat as you wish to have this great body."[52] Thus, the reporter exoticized this woman's beauty by implying that it required no work or discipline, that it had a natural excessiveness that upset the norms of a more contained femininity associated with modeling. The organizers and contestants seem to use the banter of the media to their advantage, since they do not take the contest that seriously in the first place.

The contest takes place at the Saara market in the center of Rio de Janeiro during a normal weekday, attracting the attention of hundreds of workers and shoppers going about their day. The contestants parade in bikinis, but they also wear short shorts, leopard prints, lingerie, and similar clothing that would never be considered appropriate in a traditional beauty pageant. Additionally, they do not simply walk down the makeshift runway: they dance *pagode* and *funk* (musical styles associated with the working class), they toss their hair around dramatically, and some even crawl on their hands and knees. The audience responds to these over-the-top performances with enthusiasm, by hooting loudly and hollering sexual compliments, and the contestants flirt back. The contestants who are eliminated sometimes make a scene as they leave, complaining to the cameras that they are obviously more beautiful than the winner.[53] In short, the contest is a celebration of unapologetic sensuality, corny clothing, and outrageous behavior that the operators of a traditional pageant would dismiss as debasing, vulgar, and unsophisticated.

The affective labor performed in this working-class representation of beauty is radically different from the affect deployed in the hegemonic narratives about beauty that I previously examined. The Concrete-Roof Girl is a parody of conventional beauty pageants, replacing the flawless image of a delicate, refined femininity with an unseemly and unruly femininity that is purposefully tasteless. As noted by Laura Kipnis, it is this very tastelessness that is transgressive and powerful, because it upsets bourgeois mores regarding privacy, shame, and disgust and, thus, serves as a reminder of the excessive, grotesque materiality of the body that can never be fully contained and disciplined.[54]

I would add that this tastelessness also destabilizes the teleological time frame that imagines beauty as a form of social ascension. By grounding beauty in the immediacy of the sensual and grotesque body, the unruly sexuality of the Concrete-Roof Girl engages in an alternative politics of beauty that might perhaps approximate Edelman's call to refuse hope for the future and revel instead in the enjoyment of the present.[55] There are no objectives to the contest other than the immediate enjoyment of the event itself, and no promises of betterment and so-called "social inclusion." The immaterial forms of value produced by the contest, like the recognition of the winners, are embedded in the spatiotemporal context of the Saara market and the neighborhoods where these women live and work. It is not a form of value that can in turn generate more capital and surplus value, constantly demanding more labor from them. The contest does not completely reject hope altogether, however, because it constructs a space where queer, unruly forms of beauty emerge as alternatives to hegemonic forms of beauty. In the words of José Muñoz, the Concrete-Roof Girl generates "a kind of potentiality that is open, indeterminate, like the affective contours of hope itself."[56] Spectators enjoy the contest precisely because it is unpredictable: one never knows what the next contestant will do or wear, unlike in the traditional pageants, with their strict conventions. These contestants possess a beauty that exists for its own sake and does not require the recognition of experts to reach its potential.

HOPE AGAINST HOPE

Beauty pageants that promise a better future for participants continue to proliferate across Brazil. One of the latest iterations is the Miss Penitentiary contest, held in several women's prisons with support from the government. Its stated purpose is to "elevat[e] the self-esteem of female prisoners, in order to diminish internal conflict and provide them a greater chance of becoming reintegrated within society."[57] The notion that by performing beauty these female prisoners can be reintegrated into society implies that beauty is a redemptive quality, on which not only individuals but also society as a whole must pin their hopes. This contest entailed no political engagement with the structural inequalities that landed these women in jail, such as the lack of economic opportunity, the criminalization of small drug offenses, and the racial inequalities of the criminal justice system.

The name given to the contest by the administration of the São Paulo state penitentiary system, Rewriting the Future, invokes feminine beauty as a linchpin of future citizenship and upward mobility.[58] This hope tied to beauty is problematic not only because it reduces the value of women to their bodily capacities to perform beauty, but also because it reinforces the racialized, classed, and gendered norms that tie beauty to whiteness, sexual propriety, and gender normativity. The main problem with the narratives that promise upward mobility to poor women is that the recognition of their beauty always comes from outside—from a wealthier man who seeks to marry her, from a modeling scout who discovers her as a model, from a talent agent who evaluates her potential, or from a judge at a beauty pageant. Beauty becomes a form of capital, in other words, only as a product of its circulation within an affective economy that has been predetermined by the white male gaze that reinforces Brazil's aesthetic hierarchy.

The valorization of beauty, however, does not always foreclose political engagement. For example, beauty pageants that celebrate black beauty, organized by Afro-Brazilian associations and nongovernmental organizations that promote racial equality, usually become opportunities to articulate political positions. For example, one of the most famous Carnival parades in the city of Salvador, Ilê Aiyê, which is closely tied to candomblé and the Afro-Brazilian movement, elects a Deusa do Ébano (Ebony Goddess) every year. She is considered a representative not only of black beauty but also of the Afro-Brazilian community more generally, and thus she has to be able to communicate the political views of the movement to the world at large, defending, for example, affirmative-action policies based on race.[59] The Ebony Goddess also must perform an "authentic" blackness, by wearing traditional African dress and styling her hair in a way that revalues its natural texture.

The concern with authenticity is also manifest in Osasco's Beleza Negra (Black Beauty) contest organized in the state of São Paulo and sponsored by the Osasco prefecture's Office for Women and Racial Equality. The contest regulations required that male and female participants identify as *afro-descendentes* (descendants of Africans), that they participate in a workshop about Afro-Brazilian history before the event, and that they model traditional African garb during the contest.[60] Black beauty contests such as this explicitly try to raise political consciousness and attempt to directly challenge the beauty norms that devalue blackness. More research needs to be done on these pageants; but like the Concrete-Roof Girl contest, they perhaps represent another modality of hope—not one that is cruelly attached to political structures that reinforce aesthetic hierarchies, but rather, one that is tied to a hope "that helps escape from a script in which human existence is reduced."[61]

CHAPTER 5

The Raciology of Beauty

In 2010, several Brazilian blogs and forms of social media featured a popular meme with the title "I wasn't ugly, I was poor." The meme featured before and after pictures of several American and Brazilian celebrities, showcasing their transformations into more beautiful people as they gained access to plastic surgeries, hair treatments, teeth straightening procedures, and other cosmetic treatments. The meme seemed to suggest that beautification is the clearest marker of class mobility, indexing a body's movement from poverty to riches, and from anonymity to superstardom. Beautification was also intricately interwoven with gender and race, since most of the celebrities showcased in the meme were women, and many of them were portrayed as becoming beautiful because they lost weight or because they lost racialized characteristics such as Afro-textured hair or a wide nose.

One celebrity frequently portrayed was the black news anchor and journalist Glória Maria, with an old "before" picture portraying her with an Afro, and a recent "after" picture portraying her with flowing straight hair. One blogger joked that in the "before" picture, she could be confused with the male soccer player Pelé, and another one superimposed the "before" face on the body of an African woman wearing traditional ethnic garb. Glória Maria, in other words, was portrayed as undesirable, queerly masculine, and primitive before conforming to recognizably beautiful gender and racial norms. The meme was meant to surprise its audience by playing on the contrast between a celebrity's familiar face, as seen on television or in magazines, and an unfamiliar, hidden past that the public eye had not been aware of or had long forgotten. The blogs that reposted this meme thus reveled in the Internet's ability to deconstruct the positive public image that had been carefully crafted by these celebrities.

There is more to this meme, however, than simply tearing celebrities down from their pedestals. It also reaffirms the widespread belief in Brazilian society that cosmetic practices can indeed transform a common, flawed human being into someone admired and coveted by others. Glória Maria's natural hair was a sign of that commonness, one that needed to be shed for her to become famous. Virginia Blum has argued that celebrities represent idealized versions of our own bodies—we venerate stars for their beauty and their ability to shape-shift through makeup, dress, or surgery, and contemporary culture's obsession with them is an indicator of a deep-seated identification with them. When we criticize celebrities for having gone too far in terms of surgery, as in the case of Michael Jackson, there is a thrilling aspect to unmasking their humanity and seeing how they have mismanaged their promise.[1]

The "I wasn't ugly, I was poor" meme, however, used Michael Jackson as the punch line of the entire meme, since you encountered him after scrolling to the end of the page, where instead of contrasting Michael Jackson to his younger self, the meme compared him to a chimpanzee from the film *Planet of the Apes*. The joke relied on the audience's preconscious, affective association between blackness and apelike qualities—significantly, the Portuguese word for ape or monkey, *macaco,* does not simply reference a type of animal in Brazil but is also a common racial epithet directed at black Brazilians. Kathy Davis points out that this comparison of Michael Jackson to an ape, which has been circulating on the Internet at least since 2001, shows how old biopolitical notions, such as the one that equates Africans to primates within the Great Chain of Being, can resurface in contemporary popular culture.[2] It is only in the Brazilian context, however, that this image became part of the larger "I wasn't ugly, I was poor" meme and seemed to suggest that the only difference between Michael Jackson and an ape are practices of beautification like plastic surgery, which allowed him to shape-shift out of his own race and into celebrity. Racialized forms of affect cannot be separated from the biopolitics of beauty in Brazil.

Plastic surgery and other rituals of beautification are raciological practices within the Brazilian imaginary. In other words, beautification is understood as a science of racial improvement that can create a more harmonious and aesthetically pleasing "Brazilian race," thus resurrect-ing old eugenics discourses in the contemporary context. I believe that we must look not only at medical discourses themselves to trace how race becomes a biopolitical object of intervention, but also at the ways that race circulates as a form of affect within larger popular culture, such as in the meme I just analyzed. The raciology of beauty gains trac-tion in the Brazilian context because it has biopolitical and affective dimensions that reinforce each other constantly—helping explain why raciologies still matter in today's world. Paul Gilroy has defined raciol-ogy as the set of discourses that produce color or race as the truth of human biology, and what I find most compelling about his term is the notion that race is a fiction that is continually reconstituted in different forms, and that racial schemas need constant work to be maintained.

Gilroy believes that raciologies are currently in crisis, and is hopeful that raciologies will wither away as more accurate scientific approaches to the body are developed.[3] I am less optimistic. The biopolitical dis-courses about race have an uncanny way of refashioning themselves into new shapes; and as Priscilla Wald argues, the same scientists who claim that race has no scientific basis can end up subtly perpetuating its inequi-ties through scientific narratives that are inadvertently interwoven with racialist thought.[4] Donna Haraway similarly points out that the semiot-ics of race transit promiscuously between the discourses of science, law, and industry, on the one hand, and popular images, artistic creations, and national icons, on the other.[5] Adopting Haraway's methodology, I seek to untangle the webs of meanings that produce the raciology of beauty, both affectively and biopolitically, by moving back and forth between popular culture and the medical discourse of plastic surgeons, mediating both through the insights of ethnography.

The literature about race in Brazil has brought to our attention how central aesthetic evaluations of beauty are in daily experiences of racism. For example, Robin Sheriff and Kia Caldwell, among others, have remarked that the association between blackness and ugliness constantly devalues the facial features and hair of dark-skinned individuals, forming a central aspect of their larger devaluation in society.[6] John Burdick and Donna Goldstein have explored how the aesthetic value assigned to whiteness, coupled with the hypersexualization of black bodies, affects the romantic relationships and job opportunities of dark-skinned women.[7] More recently, Elizabeth Hordge-Freeman has demonstrated that even in dark-skinned families there exists a marked preferential treatment for lighter-skinned family members, who are considered prettier.[8] I build on this literature by exploring further the architecture of racism that under-girds these aesthetic evaluations of race. Instead of focusing on racism encountered by dark-skinned Brazilians, I turn to how whiteness is expe-rienced, reproduced, medicalized, and policed by privileged, upper- and middle-class Brazilians.

Whiteness, as an unmarked racial category, needs to be more fully theorized for the Brazilian context, where lighter skin correlates strongly with class privilege, but where the national narrative of miscegenation allows even the whitest Brazilians to claim they are of mixed race. Patri-cia de Santana Pinho calls this a "white but not quite" racial construc-tion that renders whiteness unstable and inconsistent, in need of being "implicitly and carefully manipulated by individuals and groups in their ongoing microstruggles for power" rather than emerging as an explicit mark that is always visible on the body.[9] According to Liv Sovik, "The silent hypervalorization of whiteness makes sense not because domi-nant classes are uniformly white," but because any exceptions to the rule only reaffirm whiteness as a hegemonic aesthetic ideal.[10]

Among Brazilian plastic surgeons, who all belong to the upper eche-lons of society, and among their middle- and upper-class patients, white-ness is the unmarked ideal by which all bodies are measured. Whiteness, as Sheriff has pointed out, is seen as a genetic resource and a form of capital by the Brazilian middle and upper classes.[11] The raciological operations that link whiteness to beauty take two different forms. On the one hand, medical discourses about beauty provide biopolitical confir-mation of the aesthetic hierarchies that position whiteness—particularly facial characteristics—as more beautiful, even as these discourses por-tray the black body as more erotic and thus still valuable within the miscegenated nation. Biopolitics seeks to produce race as a scientific truth that can be read on bodies, and its medical concerns solidify around specific bodily parts, which then become objects of intervention. Racial-ized forms of affect, on the other hand, are more fluid forms of embodi-ment that circulate between and through bodies; and as Mel Chen argues, they blur boundaries between the human and the nonhuman, animalizing humans in queer ways.[12]

I am interested, in particular, in the ways that the concerns with beautification betray the instability of whiteness in the Brazilian con-text, both in the narratives of middle- and upper-class patients and in images from popular culture and the mass media. Whiteness emerges only in contrast with its opposite, the eroticized body of the mulatta or the feared body of the criminal, and requires constant upkeep to become a reality. To study whiteness as a fragile state, but also as one backed by powerful biopolitical claims, is to rethink how racial privilege is maintained and reproduced through Brazil's aesthetic hierarchy. Racial mattering resides in this in-between state, appearing relatively solid under certain circumstances but menacingly indeterminate and fluid in others, acquiring a viscous quality that sticks to bodies in multiple ways.[13]

THE BEAUTY OF MISCEGENATION

The concept of *miscegenação* (miscegenation) is central to Brazilian self-portrayals about the nation's identity and character. The "mixture of the three races"—white, indigenous, and black—is described in Brazilian music, literature, and popular culture as a fusion that gave origin to Brazil's unique culture and racial composition, differentiating Brazil from every other nation.[14] As I noted in chapter 1, miscegenation began to be celebrated as a positive force for the nation at the beginning of the twentieth century, in an effort by neo-Lamarckian sanitarists and eugenicists to counter the European conviction that all racially miscegenated populations were predestined to degeneration. This neo-Lamarckian science relied on a raciology that valued whiteness as a sign of healthier, fitter, and more beautiful populations, producing an aesthetic hierarchy that valued certain racial characteristics over others. The imagined eugenic future, therefore, would produce a more homogeneous nation, without as much racial variation and without ugliness.

As early as the 1930s, and with full support of the eugenicists, plastic surgery became an acceptable biopolitical tool to manage the beauty of middle- and upper-class women. Plastic surgeons were the ideal candidates to assume neo-Lamarckian objectives as their own, because theirs was a medical discipline that, like eugenics, associated people's outward, physical characteristics with individual well-being and national progress. In the 1960s, plastic surgery began to expand into the public health-care system as well, based on Ivo Pitanguy's notion that the poor, too, deserved "the right to beauty." In chapter 2, I described how Pitanguy gained the support of the state by portraying plastic surgery as a humanitarian effort, one that would not only reduce individual suffering but also lead to the betterment of society as a whole, by eliminating the physical defects associated with poverty, violence, and criminality. Pitanguy's disciples have replicated his model all over the country, opening plastic surgery services in publicly funded hospitals whose programs double as medical residencies for surgeons in training.

Ivo Pitanguy is a fascinating figure, not only because he is a household name and is admired nationwide, but also because he has carefully crafted his public persona as a philosopher and artist, as well as a man of science. He conceives of the body as a malleable canvas on which plastic surgeons can demonstrate their skill. For example, he wrote an article titled "Creativity and Plastic Surgery" praising the plastic surgeon's ability to innovate, comparing the profession to those of poets, artisans, and other artists driven by creative impulses. Pitanguy points out that the artistic limits of the plastic surgeon are imposed by the anatomy of the human body and the will of the patient, and therefore the surgeon must prepare the patient physically and psychologically before surgery, "just as the painter prepares his canvas and his paints, and the sculptor his marble."[15] His discourse is neo-Lamarckian to the extent that he conceives of the body as plastic and compliant under the influence of medical science, with beautification serving as a measure of the improvement created by the surgeon.

In the same article, Pitanguy also argues that the increase in demand for plastic surgery could be interpreted as "the search for *eugenia* [eugenesis]. . . . Several factors, such as regular sporting activity and the greater exposure of the body, [have] stimulated the quest for surgical techniques that can diminish many different deformities."[16] The pursuit of eugenic ideals through beautification is portrayed here as complementary to other aspects of leading a healthier lifestyle, which the mindful consumer-patient should make use of to eliminate dysgenic deformities. Similarly, in an interview for the newspaper *O Globo* celebrating his more than fifty years of medical practice, Pitanguy laments that members of the working class still eat and drink unhealthy foods without being aware of the consequences for their bodies, and he defends the healthy habits and medical knowledge that lead to "the eugenic sense of caring for the body."[17] For Pitanguy, beauty is a product of eugenic health, and plastic surgery plays a key role in making that beauty come to the fore even in Brazil's poor populations.

Pitanguy's use of the words *eugenesis* and *eugenics* could be interpreted as an appropriation of anachronistic terms that no longer have racialized meanings. He has repeatedly claimed, after all, that a patient should care for his own image while staying true to "his own proportions, his biotype, his race, his ethnicity, his group."[18] Brazilian plastic surgeons would never claim that their project is one of transforming an individual's race or color—they always claim that any change made to a person's physiognomy is merely meant to "harmonize" the features of patients who present discordant racial characteristics. Harmonization, however, always betrays a tendency toward whiteness, because whiteness is never pathologized as a problem to be overcome, and because it is assumed from the start to be an unmarked aesthetic ideal.

For example, the personal website of two plastic surgeons, one of whom studied with Pitanguy, explains how miscegenation produced the "Brazilian nose" and the care plastic surgeons must take in order to treat it properly:

> It is not a novelty to us Brazilians that we are the product of the combination of three basic races, and because of that it becomes so complicated to know our own *cor* [color]. . . . It is a history of unimaginable mixture among our ancestors. . . . To perform a rhinoplasty in this situation of *miscegenação* [miscegenation], the plastic surgeon must take into account the nuances of individuality and harmony in relation to the expressed desire for change. . . . A technical evaluation of the races shows that the skin of the *negro* tends to be thicker. . . . *[A]fro-descendentes* [descendants of Africans] have more delicate nasal cartilage, larger nostrils and the lack of a nasal dorsum. . . . We must preserve the facial physiognomy, the personality and the primordial ethnic characteristics.[19]

We can sense a certain tension in this discourse, one that portrays racial mixture in Brazil as pervasive, making color indeterminate, yet it also calls for respecting primordial ethnic characteristics. Black skin is portrayed as more difficult to operate on, and the black nose is pathologized as a delicate, imperfect structure that needs special care from the plastic surgeon. Since everyone is imagined as racially mixed, the surgeon's job is to harmonize the patient's nose with his or her other features, so that the nose does not harm the individuality of the patient. The very idea of harmony is reminiscent of the Freyrian description of Brazil as a nation that is exceptional because it is "constituted by harmonious racial relations,"[20] an ideology that is deployed by conservative intellectuals even today to claim that racism or racial tension does not exist in Brazil. A harmonious body, therefore, is perhaps metonymic for this biopolitical ideal of a racially harmonious nation.

The talk about harmonizing features was a constant component of plastic surgery conferences I attended, particularly when surgeons were giving a presentation about facial characteristics. Additionally, most plastic surgeons I talked to thought of miscegenation as the central engine of Brazilian difference, which made harmonization necessary in the first place. At the 2006 Meeting of the International Society of Aesthetic Plastic Surgery in Rio de Janeiro, for example, I was introduced to a group of Brazilian surgeons that was having a lively conversation after one of the panels ended. I asked these surgeons why they thought plastic surgery was so popular in their country. They all agreed that miscegenation was what gave plastic surgery so much appeal in Brazil, because it makes "white women desire the buttocks and breasts of black women," while "everyone else desires European noses," particularly *nordestinos* (northeasterners) after moving to the Southeast.[21] As I mentioned in the previous chapter, Brazilians imagine the southern regions of Brazil as whiter and more beautiful than the northern regions of the country. This national geography of beauty also shapes the aim of surgery, according to plastic surgeons: northeasterners are imagined as rural migrants who seek to become whiter through nose surgeries, while white women are imagined as approximating their bodies to the eroticized bodies of black women by enhancing their curves.

Plastic surgery, in a sense, complements the work of miscegenation by providing patients the ideal physical features of "Brazilianness" they are lacking, but it does not undo the aesthetic hierarchies that plastic surgeons also assume to be true. After all, surgeons only appreciate blackness for its sensual excess and locate its value in the lower regions of the body, reiterating the physicality for which darker-skinned Brazilians are always valued within the body politic. Facial characteristics, on the other hand, are valued when they approximate whiteness, because the face is the symbol of authority and presence in Brazilian society. The implication is that northeasterners will become upwardly mobile by getting rid of the noses that mark them as rural migrants, gaining social recognition in the process, but white women, in essence, trade respectability for black sensuality.

Dr. Mario, the chief plastic surgeon at First Federal Hospital, told me that virtuousness lies in equilibrium, such as in producing a femininity that is neither too sexy nor too demure. He gave as an example the supermodel Gisele Bündchen, whom he said benefited from her German ancestry but was nonetheless "more beautiful and feminine than German women themselves," because she walks down the catwalk with the *cadência* (swing) of mulattas—the black dancers associated with the annual Carnival. It was miscegenation, he claimed, that "made the Brazilian race a beautiful race." For Dr. Mario, then, Bündchen represents an ideal hybridity, a whiteness slightly tinged by the sensuality of blackness, perceptible only in her movements and the sway of her hips—a learned behavior that connects her to the mulatta only through this cultural practice, not in a biological sense.

Dr. Mario could have chosen many Brazilian celebrities who are brunettes and have slightly dark skin, like Camila Pitanga or Juliana Paes, to exult the value of Brazilian hybridity, and I think it is telling that he chose a supermodel of clear Germanic descent instead, betraying a desire for whiteness as the ultimate aesthetic ideal. On a different day, while his medical residents were performing a liposuction on a light-skinned woman who had complained of fat deposits on her hips, known as *culote,* Dr. Mario told me that this was a "typical aesthetic problem of the Brazilian race," characterized as it was by miscegenation. He clearly medicalized this woman's wide hips as a problem of too much racial hybridity—an excessive physicality that needed to be extracted from the body. Miscegenation is an asset for people like Bündchen, where traces of blackness can be sensual; but it can become a liability for women when blackness veers off into an improper hypersexuality or into bodily excess.

Why, then, compare Gisele Bündchen to a mulatta? As Natasha Pravaz has argued, mulattas are icons of racial mixture in Brazil because they are black but relatively light-skinned, and their *cadência* (swing) is naturalized as an innate ability emerging from their bodies.[22] The dancing body of the Carnival mulatta is an emblem of national celebration and serves as a centerpiece for each samba school association—organizations that compete against one another to put together the most extravagant floats, costumes, and choreography during the yearly Carnival parade. Even though mulattas have been associated with Carnival since the 1930s, when Afro-Brazilian cultural expressions like samba were adopted as symbols of national culture, the standardization of the samba school parades beginning in the early 1970s for televised presentations has transformed mulattas into spectacles for cultural education and touristic consumption.[23]

Every year, the Globo network chooses a mulatta as the Globeleza (Globo queen), who is then showcased dancing samba nearly nude, with just glitter or paint decorating her body, in the television vignettes that open each parade. It is the only time of the year that black beauty takes center stage in mainstream media, but it is also a beauty valued merely for its physicality and sensuality, exemplified by the Globeleza's lack of clothing and her silence in every vignette.[24] It is also a celebration of blackness that is quickly disappearing, as this vignette gets replaced with more sanitized versions that portray lighter-skinned women, or as white female celebrities become the main dancers for wealthy samba schools, relegating black dancers to lesser roles—Robin Sheriff has described this as the "theft of Carnival" from the poor.[25] The rest of the year, mulattas represent a sexual availability that is dangerous and improper, and they largely disappear from mainstream media.[26] This is the time when Bündchen triumphantly dominates television, as the main exponent of the white beauty that is usually celebrated, and her presence and voice are ubiquitous in Brazilian ads for every product imaginable, including the body itself.

To give a brief example, a news article titled "The Formula for the Perfect Legs" portrays Bündchen's full body as she lies fully clothed on a bed, her legs elegantly displayed across the page, evidently representing an ideal to aspire to. Three plastic surgeons interviewed for the piece agree that Brazilian models like Bündchen display the perfect "harmony between legs and hips," that this is a beauty found only in "the South of the country, where most of our international models come from, [and that] it does not reflect the mixture of the races that is so characteristic of Brazil."[27] Instead, owing to miscegenation, most Brazilian women have thighs that are too thick or hips that are too wide and which suffer from *culote*. The surgeons recommend liposculpture to redistribute the fat more properly—liposuction is frequently portrayed as one way to discipline the excessiveness of the body. This article is particularly pessimistic about miscegenation and its effect on Brazilian female bodies: "To have those kinds of legs, you have to be born with them," one surgeon remarks.

Other news articles are a little more celebratory. One portrays buttocks implants as providing curves to foreign women who lack sensuality, "imitating the glutes of those Brazilian women . . . privileged by racial miscegenation."[28] An article in the magazine *Plástica e Beleza* (Plastic Surgery and Beauty), quotes a surgeon who claims, "The butt of the Brazilian woman is, without a doubt, the most successful one around the world. . . . In Brazil, we have that marvelous mixture of races, which made the butt of Brazilian women . . . firmer and more projected, which does not happen in American or European women. . . . When one thinks of Brazil, especially abroad, they imagine black women with large butts, which has become a national standard."[29] The buttocks are racialized as a desirable quality that is popular not only in Brazil but also around the globe—a symbol of the national femininity that foreigners consume, as embodied by the Carnival mulatta. Although the article lauds the Brazilian butt, it also positions this type of beauty as one "for export" that does not always correspond with national desires, and it points out that liposuction and breast implants are much more popular surgical procedures than buttocks implants. As Jennifer Manthei notes, this association of black women and mulattas with touristic and foreign consumption reaffirms the local preference for whiteness.[30]

While the beauty of the body seems to result from containing but not entirely erasing blackness, this ambivalence disappears when surgeons are talking about facial features. Plastic surgeons assume Caucasian facial features are ideal, but usually they are careful to point out that they do not seek to whiten patients, only to "soften" the patient's features so that they are more harmonious in relation to the rest of the face. Surgeons are also particularly proud of their ability to transform the face, and they perceive it as an aspect of their work that is more important and more delicate than any of the surgeries they perform on the body. When I asked a medical resident specializing in plastic surgery why his medical specialty was growing so quickly in Brazil, he answered that it had to do with the plastic surgeon's ability to improve the face, not the body: "The mixture of races in Brazil left a lot of people with the wrong nose or ear. That is why people do surgery, to look like those beautiful people that mixed less, like [blonde models] Gisele Bündchen and Daniella Cicarelli. Sometimes whole families undergo nose surgery so that they do not have their father's nose."

This medical resident understood miscegenation as a process that sometimes went awry, producing mismatched characteristics on the face. Individuals and families had to seek surgery to erase traces of this inappropriate racialization that distances them from beauty. Plastic surgery is able to correct such errors and provide people with features that are representative of less racial mixture, such as those of the ubiquitous Bündchen. For plastic surgeons, Bündchen is a source of national pride because she can borrow from the mulatta's sensuality while remaining an antidote to her. She keeps reappearing in the discourse of plastic surgeons because she is an icon of white femininity, someone relatively distant from the hypersexual image of the mulatta, yet still a sex symbol who dominates billboards, ads, and magazine covers across Brazil. Her body is consumed abroad in a way unlike the manner in which the body of the mulatta is consumed. Her thin body is associated not with excess but with discipline. Her German ancestry becomes a symbol of how miscegenation can go right and produce a white, unmarked beauty that transcends national borders, without sexualizing the nation in an inappropriate way.

OF SAMBA QUEENS AND CRIMINALS

With their marble entranceways and designer furnishings, the private clinics where upper- and middle-class patients undergo plastic surgery look like five-star hotels. I was introduced to Lygia at one of these clinics by her plastic surgeon, who described her as one of his most loyal customers. Lygia had undergone four aesthetic surgeries with him over the course of the last twenty years, and was now preparing to undergo a fifth surgery. At the time we spoke, Lygia was fifty-nine years old and described herself as a business owner and housewife living in the affluent Zona Sul (South Zone) of Rio de Janeiro. As I explained to her what my research was about, she seemed taken aback by my account that aesthetic surgeries were being performed in public hospitals. In Lygia's mind, my mention of lower-income women worried about their appearance immediately conjured up images of women in samba schools, particularly mulattas. In her view, those women were naturally endowed with good bodies, and even doing exercise, much less plastic surgery, seemed redundant: "The women in samba schools want the perfect body and work out a lot. . . . But mulattas become too muscular when they work out. They already have bodies like that naturally and then end up with six-pack abs and legs that are too muscular; it's not pretty. People who are dark-skinned cannot get plastic surgery anyway, right? They end up with keloids; the result is not as good." She then contrasted her own body, which she said always needed "a lot of care," with the naturally fit bodies of mulattas.

What surprised me about Lygia's rejection of plastic surgery for the poor was the fact that she herself had not come from wealth. She and her husband had built their business from the ground up, starting with a single juice bar at Copacabana beach, then expanding their business until they owned several locations across the neighborhood. I wondered whether her upward mobility had something to do with her commitment to surgically altering her body. Lygia was not very light-skinned, and she was short and stocky and, thus, did not "look the part" compared to the taller, thin, white socialites of Rio de Janeiro's posh South Zone. The nose job, face-lift, liposuction, and breast lift she had undergone over the last two decades were all part of a project of self-improvement that seemed to use plastic surgery as a way to approximate her own body to the whiter, more distinguished body she desired. The notion that working-class women were getting cheap or free aesthetic surgeries in public hospitals disturbed Lygia, because it seemed to belie her perception that her body was perfectible through surgery in a way that poorer, darker bodies were not. She also mentioned keloids (a type of scarring that is medically constructed as more common in people of African descent) as a medical reason why people with darker skin should not get plastic surgery in any case—as if aesthetic surgery itself had been developed for bodies like hers, not other types of bodies.

Lygia's reaction was common among my upper- and middle-class interviewees, who embraced the portrayal of plastic surgeons as humanitarians who performed altruistic reconstructive surgeries in public hospitals on burn victims and people with deformities, while performing aesthetic surgeries on the wealthy. As the anthropologist Teresa Caldeira argues, the consumption of luxury items by the working class is perceived as abhorrent and wasteful by the upper classes, since ultimately it threatens the boundaries between social classes that consumption is supposed to provide.[31] The affective capital provided by plastic surgery is also meant to reinscribe racial differences that the upper and middle classes believe set them apart, and it is not supposed to be readily accessible to everyone.

We can see a contradiction, therefore, between plastic surgeons who believe that their medical discipline is a form of racial improvement for poor and wealthy alike, and the upper- and middle-class patients who believe that aesthetic plastic surgery, as a luxury item, is a marker of distinction and whiteness. The biopolitical project of plastic surgery is not simply internalized by Brazilian patients, but rather is refracted through forms of affect that racialize bodies in more ways than one. While plastic surgeons utilize the iconic figure of the samba school queen, usually imagined as a mulatta, to indicate the sensual potential of all Brazilian women, for women like Lygia the samba school queens had naturally muscular bodies that served as a counterpoint to their own bodies, perfectible through surgery. Whiteness is simultaneously more desirable and more fragile in the nonmedical discourse, always seeking to distance itself from marked racial identities and to emerge as the unmarked ideal. There is always the possibility, however, that this process will go wrong, that it will go in the opposite direction.

Take, for example, the caricature of a Carnival samba queen in figure 9, which circulated widely on Facebook, and which, like Lygia, critiques the fact that these women are becoming more and more muscular every year. Even though the caricature portrays a relatively light-skinned samba queen—perhaps a reference to and critique of female white celebrities who have recently assumed that role within samba schools—it still racializes her by suggesting that her physicality is a dangerous devolution into apelike characteristics. Although the orange color of the primate in the last frame indicates an orangutan, its fierce visage and imposing size suggest a gorilla—an implicit blackness that associates

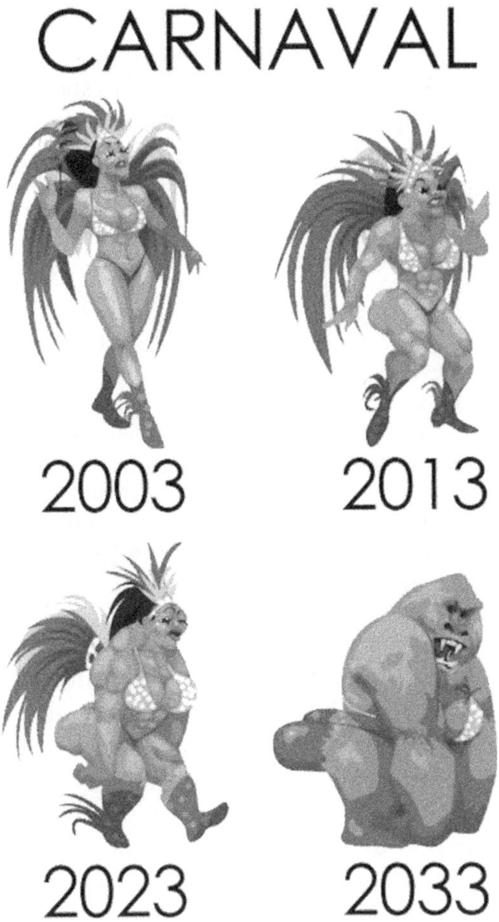

FIG 9. Meme circulating on the Internet portraying a racialized caricature of a samba queen.

the descent into animality with racial inferiority. Not only does the samba queen become more muscular in every frame, but also her buttocks and breasts become obscenely large, indicating a body marked by its excessive physicality and sensuality. The relative whiteness of the samba school queen is negated by the sexualization and animalization of her body, which, as Anne McClintock and Mel Chen argue, refer to old forms of racist iconography that easily travel between bodies.[32]

In contrast to this excessive, queer, nonwhite body, the white upper-class female body is affectively constructed as a more proper, decorous, and contained body. This became clear to me in an interview with Elisa, a fifty-two-year-old business administrator from Rio de Janeiro, who prided herself on the meticulous care she had taken of her body since she was fifteen. She religiously worked out at the gym two hours every morning before heading to work, she ate only healthy food to stay thin, and she had undergone four plastic surgeries so far: she had her nose and ears done when she was thirty, she got silicone breast implants at thirty-nine, and she had a face-lift at fifty-one.

Elisa contrasted her own quest for beauty with the beauty of women from the *morro* (hillside shantytown, favela):

> Beauty is imposing itself in a pathological, unhealthy way everywhere. . . . Even Brazilians with little culture want to become beautiful, and a *pretinha* [black girl] from the *morro* believes she can become a model [and] use beauty as a passport. But how many can achieve that in a country of 180 million people? In the *morro* they all have large buttocks, typical of Brazilian culture. . . . If a woman from the *morro* climbs [the social ladder] she will get plastic surgery. No samba school queen has a natural body, even though the black woman has a beautiful body. Carla Perez, for example: now she is another person. She took out that *nariz de crioulo* [nigger nose] and she got liposuction; now she even has her own aesthetic clinic.

In Elisa's eyes, the natural body of the black woman might be beautiful, but it is still marked by its excessive qualities, such as large buttocks—she critiqued the belief that this body could provide upward mobility, considering it an unrealistic expectation. While Elisa portrayed her own surgeries as a necessary form of maintenance that kept her body "up to date," she considered surgery among the poor to be pathological or unhealthy, unless it occurred after they had become wealthy. It is significant that she chose Carla Perez, a celebrity born in poverty but who rose to fame as part of a musical dance troupe, and who is blonde and relatively light-skinned, as the example of someone who could become another person through plastic surgery. The liposuction and nose surgery that Perez underwent had, in Elisa's eyes, sculpted that body in particular ways, subduing a blackness tied to poverty that manifested itself in excessive curves and an unaesthetic nose racialized as nonwhite. Her use of the epithet *crioulo* to describe Carla's nose is indicative of the ways that race is viscous and attaches itself to the body no matter its skin color—Carla can have a *nariz de crioulo* without being a *crioulo*.[33]

Elisa saw the favelas in Rio de Janeiro as producing more ugliness than beauty in the city, owing to the violence and criminality she believed they unleashed on the middle class. She told me that living in Rio de Janeiro was like "living in a civil war," and that all the fear and stress caused by crime ended up aging people prematurely. Her doctor could not keep up with the great demand for plastic surgery caused by all this stress and by the inability to enjoy life. She prided herself, however, on following the recommendation of her son's therapist and taking him to soccer games in the Maracanã Stadium in order to combat the panic disorder he suffered from. She and the psychotherapist hoped that exposing the child to men from the favelas would reduce his fear of crime, since it was clear to Elisa that all those male spectators at the soccer stadium were *marginais* (criminals)—it was "visible on their face[s]," she remarked. Elisa, in other words, understood the beauty of her own white body as threatened by the darker-skinned bodies from the favelas, crafting an affective dichotomy between white beauty and criminality.

This belief that beautification is a corrective to the city's violence is widespread in Brazil's mass media. An article in the magazine *Época* on the fear caused by crime, for example, recommended exercise as a way to fight fear. The article argued that "a healthy body gives one the sensation of being better prepared" against crime, despite suggesting earlier that civilians should never react to a robbery and should never attempt to face the ruthless violence in Brazil.[34] Similarly, an advertisement for the International Conference on Aesthetics that would take place in Rio de Janeiro in 2006, whose purpose was to publicize the latest innovations in cosmetics, dieting, and aesthetic treatments, also made mention of crime as the mirror opposite of having a beautiful body. A person's very happiness, the advertisement asserted, depends on being able to counter the "stress caused . . . [in] Brazil, by the fear of violence" with adequate lifestyle choices that produce a healthy, fit body and a general sense of well-being.[35] Exercise and other beautification practices work here as clear class and racial markers, determining which bodies are dangerous and inharmonious, and which bodies are perfectible.

Middle- and upper-class Brazilians discipline their bodies through surgery not only in an effort to mark their bodies as distinct from darker-skinned bodies but also to remove any facial features that might mark them as nonwhite. For example, Rosa, a fifty-one-year-old divorcee who described herself as independently wealthy and who came from a family of Lebanese immigrants, told me she went through her first plastic surgery when she was only fifteen years old. The nose surgery had been a present from her father, who suggested the surgery in the first place. She underwent the surgery in São Paulo at the same time as two of her female cousins, both of whom had "ugly noses" like her. All of the women in her family went through the same surgery at one time or another, but not the men. She admitted she had gotten the surgery without thinking, as opposed to her two subsequent plastic surgeries as an adult.

She now believed the surgery was necessary for her and the women in her family to meet the *padrão de beleza nacional* (national beauty standard). In her opinion, however, there are two very different beauty standards in Brazil:

> You hear a lot about the *padrão* [standard]—it's that sensual, big-breasted woman; but it has nothing to do with me. . . . You have really two [standards], first the curvy mulatta, a standard for export. Women enlarge their buttocks and their breasts, but it's losing one's good sense. You also have men who like the thinner, leaner woman. Young girls go after the curvy ideal[,] . . . but they are looking for standards that are not theirs. It's crazy. We have somewhat lost the good sense of following your own beauty standard.

Rosa clearly distinguished between a beauty standard embodied by the curvy, excessive mulatta, but which "has nothing to do" with her, and a thinner, contained standard of beauty that she associated with a more refined taste. The surgery was necessary for her to meet a standard that she clearly understood as white, in contrast to the nonwhite beauty of the mulatta.

If we simply followed Bourdieu, we would argue that Rosa embraced notions of good and bad taste with the purpose of naturalizing social differences through consumption, inscribing forms of cultural capital on the body itself.[36] This would not, however, fully explain why Rosa operationalized race as a way to create distance between herself and others. Rosa critiqued young girls who had lost the sense that they could set their own standards of beauty, seemingly unaware of the inherent contradiction in claiming that mulattas are not to be emulated, while her own ethnic nose, betraying her Lebanese background, had to be reshaped. It is not simply that notions of taste are transmitted in the field of social relations, but that a form of racialized affect accumulates on bodies and assigns value to specific features while devaluing others. There is a specific history of racialization that disparages Arab ethnicities in the Brazilian public sphere,[37] and which probably influenced the decision in Rosa's family to surgically alter noses that would mark the women of the family as non-Brazilian.

If it is women who more frequently undergo these surgeries to eliminate familial imperfections, it is because their perceived beauty is considered a form of capital that makes them marriageable. Valuing women for their physical characteristics also reduces them to their reproductive potential. It is significant that Rosa's nose surgery was a present given to her on her fifteenth birthday, the age understood as the point when a girl enters womanhood. Surgery reaffirmed Rosa's whiteness at an affective, preconscious level, but it was a fragile whiteness always haunted by the viscosity of race and the possibility that Rosa herself might be somehow marked as nonwhite. In Latin America, as Elizabeth Roberts has argued, whiteness is a manifold quality that encompasses education, cleanliness, language, and appearance, precisely because race is more malleable and so intricately imbricated with notions of class.[38] I would add that whiteness, as an aspirational quality, is a racialized form of affect that slowly accumulates on subjects through certain practices of bodily cultivation.

THE NEGROID NOSE AND OTHER "PRIMITIVE FEATURES"

The Brazilian raciology of beauty simultaneously deploys biopolitical discourses and latches on to racialized forms of affect, producing a body that is both solid and fluid, as well as viscous with signification. The clearest instance where this happens is with facial structures; in the case of the nose, patients and plastic surgeons have very different conceptions of why noses matter, but they agree on the fact that noses require surgical intervention. As Rosa's story exemplifies, discourses surrounding the nose—a body part particularly subject to racialization—also make the idealization of whiteness most evident.

As a biopolitical discourse, plastic surgery has developed a complex diagnosis regarding what surgeons call the *nariz negroide,* or "negroid nose." Although the term is applied unevenly to patients, depending on skin color and other characteristics racialized as nonwhite, the negroid nose solidifies the reality of racial difference within medical discourse. These somewhat rigid biopolitical norms can be contrasted with the more fluid affects regarding *traços finos,* or "fine features," that circulate within both popular discourses and mass media, and which seem at first glance to be somewhat disconnected from race since they are promiscuously applied to people of all skin colors. The desirability of fine features, however, acquires affective significance only in relation to the devaluation of features racialized as nonwhite, such as the *nariz achatado* (flattened nose). Doctors alternate between these medical and non-medical terms used for facial features, at times deciding to exhibit their medical knowledge regarding the racialized body, and at other times employing the more subtle terms that graft onto a wide variety of meanings more easily. The translation between the two modes of racialization, biopolitical and affective, reveals the ways race transits between spaces and how it is anchored in different sets of discourses that render it true for both patients and doctors.

Plastic surgery, as a medical discipline, atomizes body parts into separate units, distinguishing skin color from other racialized characteristics. I first heard the term *negroid nose* from Dr. Mario at First Federal Hospital, and what surprised me the most was that he was applying it to a teenage girl who was not very dark-skinned. As two of the medical residents operated on her, under the supervision of Dr. Mario, I asked him why this girl, Bianca, needed surgery. For my benefit and the benefit of his students, he replied, "This girl has the typical Brazilian beauty, except for the nose. She is *morena* [brown], a product of miscegenation. She wanted to correct not only the shape but also reduce the width of the nostrils[,] . . . but it would create a scar and appear artificial. The negroid nose is very common in the Brazilian race." This was not the only time that I saw plastic surgeons classify patients as *morenos* (brown) or *brancos* (white) and then justify nose surgery by arguing that these patients had a nose that was incompatible with their skin color.

The key to understanding this apparent contradiction is the central role that plastic surgeons give to miscegenation, as the engine of racial difference in Brazil. According to Dr. Mario, Bianca was *morena* (brown) and, thus, already an emblem of the miscegenation that had created a new, racially mixed population. This brownness is beautiful to the surgeon, as the ideal midpoint between black and white. Bianca's nose, however, was a medical problem in need of surgical correction. Despite portraying it as a common characteristic of the "Brazilian race," the surgeon interpreted the negroid nose not as an aspect of hybrid beauty but as a distortion that darkened and diminished Bianca's face unnecessarily. Dr. Mario was thus able to simultaneously devalue black facial characteristics as unaesthetic and value miscegenation as a generally positive force, whose small mistakes or deviations can be corrected by plastic surgery.

When I talked to Bianca's mother, she used not the medical term *negroid nose* but the more colloquial *nariz achatado* (flattened nose), considered aesthetically unpleasing and inferior to thinner and pointier noses. Bianca's mother had brought her teenage daughter in for surgery because Bianca had complained several times of being made fun of at school for her wide nose, and her mother believed that the "right" nose would provide her with better opportunities in the future. Neither Bianca nor her mother identified as *negra* (black), and thus the surgeon seemed careful to use the colloquial language around them to avoid offending them. As Robin Sheriff argues, the term *negro* can be considered an insult unless used as a term of endearment by family members or close friends, and most people prefer to describe a dark-skinned acquaintance as *moreno* or *morena* (brown), since it is the more polite term to use.[39] Similarly, surgeons use disclaimers or invent other terms to blunt the racism of the term *negroid nose* on their websites and in other promotional material, demonstrating that they are careful to translate their atomizing medical knowledge into more fluid racial terms.

For example, an otolaryngologist who specializes in nose jobs has a website that lists *negroid, Oriental*, and *Caucasian* as three types of noses that exist in the human race, but he points out that the "miscegenated nose" is the most common type in Brazil. When he begins to describe the problems of the miscegenated nose, however, he lists the same issues he found in the negroid nose, such as the thick skin and the elongated nostrils that make it a particularly difficult nose to operate on.[40] Another website, advertising the work of two plastic surgeons, points out that "there is no such thing as an ugly nose, just one that is in disharmony with the face," and that the surgical correction of the negroid nose is thus based on patients' complaints, not on any "prejudice against *negros* [blacks] or *mestiços* [mestizos]." The website assures its readers that the diversity of Brazilian features is beautiful, but it also lists the surgical techniques available for making noses thinner and pointier.[41]

When surgeons speak to one another at conferences or via published papers, there is less ambivalence about the undesirability of the negroid nose or its specificity as a Brazilian malaise. At an aesthetic medicine conference in Rio de Janeiro, a white surgeon from the city of Salvador presented a paper on the negroid nose, portraying it as a medical challenge that requires special knowledge. The surgical correction of the negroid nose, he claimed, was becoming more common in Brazil as the races continued to mix, and as "blacks became assimilated into the middle class." He assumed, in other words, that nose surgery would accompany the upward mobility of his dark-skinned patients. As the principal instructor for a course on nose surgeries at the Federal University of Bahia—widely considered the state with the largest percentage of Afro-Brazilians in the nation—he had plenty of dark-skinned patients on which to practice new techniques for reshaping the cartilage structure that gives a nose its overall shape. At several points, he contrasted the negroid nose with the more suitable Caucasian nose, which he considered easier to operate on, but he emphasized that his surgery would not change a patient's ethnic characteristics.

At another conference, a surgeon was more explicit about the need to reassure patients that a nose surgery would "preserve racial symmetry and only correct facial asymmetries." The patient would be unhappy, he explained, if he or she ended up with a Michael Jackson nose that was too small, so the surgeon had to attempt to make a thinner nose without resorting to the techniques available for "Anglo-Saxon noses." At the several lectures I heard on the negroid nose, all speakers assumed that it was a particularly stable object of analysis that acquired meaning, and required a special type of intervention, only in relation to the more standard white nose.

Plastic surgery, like other biopolitical discourses, attempts to produce an objective analysis of the human body, flattening or pigeonholing certain bodily differences while simultaneously emphasizing others, in the effort to create discrete racial groups. In a paper published by surgeons from the Federal University of São Paulo, the authors attempt to reconcile the standardized, impartial parameters that are needed to make correct diagnoses with the "accentuated anatomical variations [of noses], due to the great racial miscegenation" that exists in Brazil.[42] These surgeons resort to anthropometry—the scientific measurement of the body[43]—in order to conduct a detailed study of eleven female patients diagnosed with negroid noses at the university's hospital. Of these patients, two are described as having *cor branca* (white color), five as having *cor parda* (brown color), and four as having *cor negra* (black color), confirming that color is indeed considered independent from the condition known as the negroid nose. The article explains that nine ideal anthropometric standards (most of them angle measurements) were developed by the surgeons, who analyzed enlarged digital photographs of all eleven patients, taken from three different perspectives before and after the surgery.

The patient whose photographs were chosen to illustrate these nine archetypal measurements in the published article, however, is a dark-skinned woman probably classified as black in the study. Placed to the left of each of her photographs are simple illustrations that resemble old raciological depictions of black inferiority, owing to the way they exaggerate the racial features depicted, such as the nose, eyes, and lips. This patient is never shown as having received the surgery—she seems to

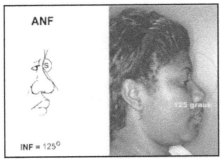

INF = 125°

Figura 6 - Ângulo Nasofrontal.

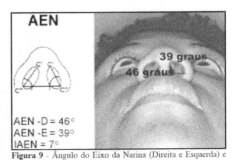

AEN -D = 46°
AEN -E = 39°
IAEN = 7°

Figura 9 - Ângulo do Eixo da Narina (Direita e Esquerda) e
Índice de Assimetria dos Eixos das Narinas.

FIG 10. Prototypical measurements of the "negroid nose," published in *Acta Cirurgica Brasileira*. Photo courtesy of Bernardo Hochman's family.

have been beyond redemption. Since her body is not a perfectible one, and instead epitomizes a medical condition, it thus serves as medical diagnostic tool (see fig. 10).

In contrast to this body diagnosed as inadequate, a lighter-skinned patient is represented in before-and-after photographs at the end of the article (fig. 11) as an instance of the successful transformation from a nonblack patient with an inaccurate negroid nose into an ideal mixed-race woman. The model patient who is to be harmonized by plastic surgery is imagined as one who has already benefited from miscegenation and can, thus, meet the plastic surgeon halfway in his fantasy of whitening the nation through surgery.

The raciology of beauty gains authority from scientific claims such as these, but it seems impractical for plastic surgeons to always rely on detailed anthropometric measurements to tell them which bodies to operate on, as well as unlikely that they would do so. In their day-to-day interactions with patients, surgeons rely instead on blurrier notions, such as their own instincts, to diagnose and treat ugliness. For example, in a book showcasing the "vision" of nine plastic surgeons, one of them argues that while popular culture might produce certain exaggerated, inadequate perceptions of beauty, the surgeon's instinct can interpret correctly what is truly beautiful:

> Our instincts know how to recognize and admire beauty as that which best performs a given function. Teeth that are white and well aligned are "beautiful" because they do not possess any dental cavities or periodontal diseases, and chew better—providing better function. Noses that are too small or too big are "ugly" because they do not allow normal breathing . . . and in most

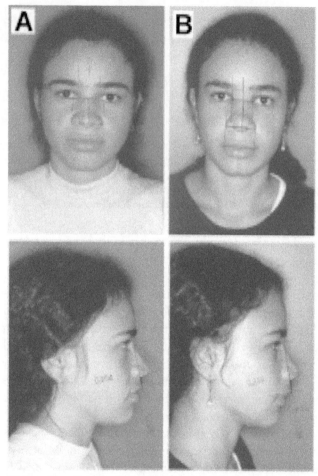

Figura 12 - Comparação de fotogrametrias nasais computa-
dorizadas (posição anterior e de perfil direito). A - pré-operatório;
B - pós-operatório.

FIG 11. A patient whose "negroid nose" has been corrected through
surgery, portrayed in *Acta Cirurgica Brasileira*. Photo courtesy of
Bernardo Hochman's family.

cases they are associated with deviations of the septum and hypertrophy of
the nasal conches—providing bad function. Breasts of adequate proportions,
round and without flaccidity are associated with a predominance of glandu-
lar tissue over adipose tissue, destining them for lactation . . . —we judge
them to be "beautiful." By these examples, we conclude that "the beautiful
is good, and the good is beautiful."[44]

In this narrative, the aesthetic preferences for whiter teeth, perfect noses, and nonflaccid breasts are stripped of any classed, raced, or gendered power dynamics that might underlie taste. Instead, the body is portrayed as visibly manifesting its state of health through beauty and ugliness, which the clinical gaze can then translate into objective medical diagnoses.

Similarly, in an article in *Veja* magazine titled "Beauty: Is Perfection Possible?" ten plastic surgeons answer the question of whether there are universal bodily proportions that link beauty to the evolution of the human species. The article sums up their conclusions as follows: "in all eras" of human history, the ideal woman possesses "wide hips and full breasts," representing her capacity to "procreate and feed healthy children," while her "*traços finos*" (fine features) are indicative of "fertility and youthfulness."[45] Beauty is portrayed here as a sexualized female body destined for reproduction, but which would not be considered fully feminine if it did not possess fine facial features—unavoidably associated with Caucasian features in the Brazilian imaginary (and reaffirmed through the pictures of white women used in the article).

Discourses about sex and race circulate in ways that end up naturalizing certain biological truths about the human body, confirming the surgeon's instinctive and authoritative recognition of what is good and beautiful. These discourses also produce affects that accumulate on certain turns of phrase, such as *traços finos,* giving them value even though those words offer a rather diffuse description of facial features. The notion of fine features is used in a wide variety of circumstances, from blogs that recommend certain makeup styles in order to make facial features look thinner, to ads for aesthetic clinics that recommend a wide variety of injections to produce them. The phrase can be applied not only to the nose but also to the lips, cheekbones, and chin and even to the shape of the neck—loosely lashing in physical characteristics depending on the context. It is only in contrast with features that are not thin that fine features become more explicitly racialized.

For instance, in the article "Doll Beauty," which appeared in the popular science magazine *Mente Cérebro* (Brainy mind) in 2007, beauty is described as an indicator of the "good genes" that represent superiority in the evolutionary scale. The article argues that *traços atraentes* (attractive features), such as those found in a Barbie doll, were products of human evolutionary advances, while the ugliness of *traços primitivos* (primitive features) lies in the fact that such features are legacies of "our ancestors." The article claims that the preference for blonde women in countries like Brazil, where "*morenos* [the brown-skinned people] predominate," is none other than the search for the "genetic diversity" that will "reinforce the immunological system of our offspring."[46] The primitive features portrayed as ugly, therefore, represent the opposite of the more desirable *traços finos* (fine features) and, thus, affectively align blackness with the primitive while establishing whiteness as aesthetically and biologically superior.

Finer or thinner features are also contrasted with the features of the criminal class in Brazil, which racializes patients in an understated manner and depends directly on the affective association between blackness and criminality that exists in the Brazilian imaginary. This became clear to me at the Fourteenth International Scientific Congress of Aesthetics, which took place in Rio de Janeiro in August 2006, during a special presentation about a new laser machine advertised as the latest breakthrough for treating skin imperfections, including acne, spots caused by the sun, and under-eye shadows. The doctor giving the presentation to an audience of doctors, physiotherapists, nurses, and aestheticians chose subtly racialized language to describe the benefits provided by the laser treatment:

> The face of the patient becomes homogenized and illuminated, and we recognize her as beautiful. The nose and lips appear *afinados* [thinner]. . . . With this machine, I can produce beauty from technique. One of my patients even cried, and we all got really emotional about the results. . . . The illumination transforms people's unconscious perceptions of the patient, making her less of a threat. Now everything will go well with her boyfriend or at work. . . . If the face becomes illuminated it becomes beautiful, because it is no longer a threat to the subconscious.

If the laser treatment is able to illuminate the face of the patient, it is because she was somehow darker or under a shadow before. If the treatment makes the nose and lips appear thinner, it is because the patient was not previously perceived as having fine features.

Without naming blackness directly, the presenter evokes it as a threat to beauty and thus to a person's happiness. Despite the fact that the laser machine could not really whiten the skin of potential patients, the presenter instrumentalized racialized forms of affect to capture the imagination of his audience. Trying to differentiate it from the competition, he portrayed the laser machine as capable of radically altering people's appearance and transforming their lives, and he assured us this would guarantee high profits for anyone who bought the product. No one in the audience challenged this representation of beautification as a way to banish darkness, and all applauded it instead.

RACIOLOGY AND ITS DISCONTENTS

Beatriz, a twenty-year-old middle-class college student, betrayed an anxiety about her own whiteness. She met me for an interview in one of the most exclusive malls in the neighborhood of Leblon, one of her favorite places to hang out. She commented that typical Brazilian beauty might be the "mixture of colors" found in the mulatta and her "big behind," but that she would never want that for herself. Instead, she aspired to be like the Brazilian supermodels Gisele Bündchen and Daniela Sarahyba, and implied that, like her, these women were not the product of any mixture but were simply white. She said she admired the bodies of runway models, whom she described as thin and *enxutos* (contained).

Beatriz seemed confident of her beauty now, since her ear surgery, but she confessed that she had once been very insecure. When she was younger, her schoolmates had taunted her because of her protruding ears, giving her the cruel nickname *macaca* (ape). Beatriz did not mention the racialized aspect of her nickname, but she did tell me that she had felt her protruding ears gave her a *cara de mau,* or the "face of bad a person." She had also felt her ears gave her a deformed appearance, an appearance that belonged to someone she was not, and she had begged her parents for ear surgery. Her father had opposed the idea, however, because he had undergone the same surgery when he was only four years old and considered it a traumatic experience. Beatriz's mother, who had *also* undergone ear surgery, but as an adult, had argued that new surgical techniques could guarantee the safety and painlessness of the surgery. After Beatriz finally underwent the surgery, which was carried out by her boyfriend's father, a plastic surgeon, she loved the result. She said she might consider other surgeries when she got older, if going to the gym and dieting were not enough to have the body she desired.

If the sensual mulatta is a recurrent archetypal figure against which upper- and middle-class women contrast their beauty, the racialized criminal is the mulatta's male counterpart—a stereotype of the dangerous ugliness that is imagined as emerging from poverty. Beatriz's comment that she did not want to have the "face of a bad person" makes clear that certain facial features are highly stigmatized in Brazilian society and circulate as signifiers of poverty and criminality. In *City of Walls,* Teresa Caldeira argues that the boundaries between social classes are reinforced through discourses about bodily differences, such as the "talk of crime" that borrows from old criminological concepts to portray migrants from northeastern Brazil as having recognizable faces that mark them as potential criminals.⁴⁷ As I have suggested, the "talk of crime" intersects the "talk of beauty" through its affective construction of facial features as either innocently beautiful or suspiciously ugly.

Additionally, racial epithets like *macaca* are powerful because they rely on biopolitical histories of racism that describe people of African descent as closer to apes than humans. Mel Chen makes the case that such affective architectures of racism not only utilize the category of the animal to dehumanize racial others but also are hierarchies that are by their very nature unstable, and thus they sometimes drag down, by association, white individuals, who usually are racially unmarked.⁴⁸ Beatriz's stable class position, normative gender presentation, and white skin did not protect her from the specter of racialization accumulating on her body. Whiteness is a precarious form of affective capital that sometimes must rely on surgery to police its borders. The end result is that surgeries sometimes run in families: Beatriz inherited the need for the ear surgery that both her parents had already carried out, in the same way that all of the women in Rosa's Lebanese family were perceived as in need of surgery to correct their noses.

This raciology has not gone unchallenged in Brazil. Black feminist bloggers, in particular, have recently become more vocal about the racial injustices that are reproduced through beauty ideals. Amanda Beatriz and Clarice Fortunato Araújo, for example, have denounced the aesthetic valorization of black women who have thin noses, straight hair, and light skin as emblems of a blackness that is desirable, thus devaluing other black phenotypes.⁴⁹ Gabi Porfírio is more direct in her critique of plastic surgery in a blog post titled "Racism Cloaked as Science," where she points out the racism inherent in the term *negroid nose* and its representation as a body part that requires special intervention:

> In a society constructed on the basis of a Eurocentric standard of beauty, we couldn't expect anything else but the association of black ethnic features with bad things: "skin the color of coal," "steel wool hair," "a potato nose," etc. This makes black people unable to accept their own characteristics and makes them feel pressured to change their bodies, many times submitting themselves to dangerous and frequently painful procedures. . . . The websites of plastic surgery clinics are experts at using demeaning terminology for the noses of black people. . . . And if that terminology were not enough to hide the racism inherent in them, the noses of black people are always "difficult," "problematic": one of the great "difficulties" of plastic surgeons is confronting a rhinoplasty of the negroid nose[,] . . . while a Caucasian nose is considered relatively easy to be improved upon and almost always has "good" aesthetic and functional results.⁵⁰

I quote this at length to show that minority voices in Brazil deconstruct beauty in ways similar to what I have done in this chapter, resisting the dominant discourses that naturalize beauty as an instinctive reaction to what is good and valuable, or as an objective analysis of aesthetic superiority. Beauty, instead, should be seen a product of specific biopolitical histories and affective processes.

I cannot do justice to Brazilian black feminist interventions here, but I hope my analysis of the raciology of beauty contributes to the ongoing conversations regarding how sexism, racism, and beauty are imbricated in the Brazilian imaginary. The examination of whiteness as a process marked by instability provides an explanation of why beauty is so sticky with signification, leading to the devaluation of characteristics racialized as nonwhite even among people who identify as white.

CHAPTER 6

Cosmetic Citizens

Renata told me her story in the waiting room of one of Rio de Janeiro's teaching hospitals. In contrast to others in the boisterous room, she sat by herself in a corner, and her body language indicated that she was timid and downcast. She seemed relieved when I approached her, however, pleased that someone was willing to listen to her complaints and write them down. Nearly a year ago she had come to this same hospital for a breast lift surgery, trusting the hospital's good reputation. She had hoped to regain the firm breasts she had had when she was younger. On the day of the surgery, however, she discovered that she would be operated on by a young Colombian medical resident she had never met before, and that the surgery would only be supervised by a senior surgeon. Renata's surgery was not successful, and after the surgery she discovered that one breast was now higher than the other, and that her nipples were out of place. She also suspected that the surgery had not been carried out in a sterile environment, because she developed severe infections in the areas where she had stitches—infections that took months to heal.

Renata had considered suing the doctor who operated on her, but she discovered that her chances of winning were slim, and that even with a lawyer working pro bono she could not afford to sue: she would still need an expert medical evaluation that would cost at least thirty-five hundred reais (about a thousand U.S. dollars) to confirm that a medical error had occurred. She could not afford this on her meager salary, so Renata had demanded that the hospital pay for the medical evaluation.

They refused, offering only to redo the surgery itself for free. In the meantime, she had to cope with having deformed breasts that made her incredibly unhappy, and which she could not fix if she wanted to sue, because they were the only proof she had of the medical error of which she had been a victim. Lowering her eyes, she told me she felt ugly and undesirable—no man would want her in the state she was in. Renata had relented, and now she was back in the same hospital for a corrective surgery, this time to be carried out by the director of the residency program. She said she would not recommend this hospital to anyone, but she also felt she had been particularly unlucky. Many of her friends had had better success here, and just one other friend had been disappointed. Renata confessed that if she were offered a tummy tuck at another hospital, she might do it. Ugliness, she told me at the end of our conversation, is something that makes people deeply unhappy, and "if you are unhappy with your body, surgery is the way to go."

How do we account for Renata's belief in plastic surgery as a way to battle unhappiness, even after such an upsetting experience at the hands of plastic surgeons? Throughout this book, I have argued that beauty matters in Brazil because it is intrinsically associated with a series of promises—the hope of upward mobility, the promise of social inclusion, and the utopian possibility of a more egalitarian society. Beauty is also experienced as a rigid aesthetic hierarchy that determines which bodies have value in society, one which condenses the race, class, and gender inequalities that patients experience in their day-to-day lives. Beautification, therefore, is regarded not as a choice but as a mandate that Brazilian citizens must obey if they want to hope for a better future. Beautification, in short, is laden with powerful forms of affect, and Renata seemed to be clearly invested in this project of self-improvement, even after it disfigured her body and deeply unsettled her life.

Understanding Renata's choices as irrational, however, would position affect as the opposite of rationality—as if emotion or feeling merely clouds our better judgment. Brian Massumi warns us that this attitude toward affect simply reasserts the neoliberal myth of an autonomous subject who bases his or her decisions on rational choice and self-interest, maximizing the greater good through the market's invisible hand. Instead, we should understand all calculations of risk as relational and intersubjective, infused by affective tendencies and by complex entanglements that belie our very autonomy.[1] According to Annemarie Mol, this lack of autonomy might be particularly true in medical settings, where the ideal of free choice is celebrated but in practice is made impossible by routine situations that detract from patients' self-determination.[2] For example, Renata's decision to have her first surgery cannot be disentangled from the public trust that plastic surgeons carefully cultivate, or from the biopolitical forms of governance that provide surgeries to the poor while defining them as willing experimental subjects. After her surgery, Renata's choices were constrained by a legal system that protects surgeons more than low-income patients, by the affective relationship to her own body, and by a neoliberal logic that puts the onus of a patient's health on the patient herself, making her responsible for her own well-being. Renata's desire for surgery is perfectly reasonable in relation to the other rationalities that delimit the legal, medical, and affective possibilities that emerge from plastic surgery.

In my view, we should think of the rationality of plastic surgery not as residing within any individual but as being distributed among a field of actors with coalescing interests and attachments. Based on the work of Bruno Latour and Tim Ingold, I consider agency to be never singular, but rather as something that is distributed among a wide variety of actants that include people, bodies, materials, and things.[3] I make the case that becoming an experimental subject is less an experience of losing agency than an experience of becoming entangled in larger calculations of risk that deprioritize the health of low-income patients. Patients who willingly become experimental subjects assume the risks that surgeons, the public health-care system, and the legal system are unwilling to assume. The costs of surgery, in other words, are externalized by the medical-industrial complex by transferring these costs onto the bodies of more vulnerable actors, the working-class patients.

I call these patients "cosmetic citizens," because they are caught in a paradoxical bind between the affective promises and the biopolitical costs of surgery, since they have to take on the burden of the risks of medicalization in order to access the promise of citizenship through surgery. I do not, however, want to portray surgeons as expert puppet masters who manipulate patients into assuming those risks. That would imply that surgeons are more rational or more calculating than their patients, when in fact they, too, are driven by the affective promises of manipulating the body, and they, too, make calculations of risk that seem to go against their very interests. I illuminate the ways in which surgeons favor innovation over safeguarding their patients (particularly if a technique promises them unlimited power over the body) by focusing on the ongoing controversy regarding bioplasty, a surgical technique that has a considerable number of backers despite its long record of causing serious health problems. In a broader sense, I explore how affect complicates our understanding of rationality, and how it helps us trace the ways in which patients and their surgeons become lashed into biopolitical networks of knowledge production.

EXPERIMENTAL SETTINGS

Rio de Janeiro is a hub of national and global conferences about plastic surgery and aesthetic medicine. It is not simply Brazil's touristic appeal that attracts doctors from around the world to the city but rather the opportunity to learn about innovative beautification techniques that are not available elsewhere. At these conferences, doctors have the opportunity to listen to scientific panels, participate in training sessions, and witness live demonstrations. The biggest conference room is usually reserved for live surgeries, which take place at a nearby hospital and are simultaneously transmitted to a large screen for the audience at the conference. The doctor performing the surgery describes in detail the methods being used on the patient and comments on how these methods have the potential to replace or improve upon older techniques. After the surgery is completed, audience members watching the live feed can ask the surgeon direct questions and learn more about the technique being presented. The doctors performing these live procedures are usually respected members of the medical community who have already proven their worth by developing innovations that many other surgeons in Brazil and abroad have adopted.

A surgeon wins prestige and symbolic capital, in other words, by sharing his or her knowledge of novel surgical techniques, which usually carry the surgeon's name and are sometimes even trademarked. This prestige translates into tangible economic capital as the surgeon becomes a requested name in the conference circuit, able to charge for presentations and training sessions, and forges a recognizable name that provides him or her with additional private clientele. Moreover, if the surgeon is promoting a procedure associated with a certain laboratory product, like silicone implants, he or she can gain extra income as a stockowner or a consultant for the laboratory. In Latourian fashion, the surgeons who seem to prevail are those who have the most backers and who have lashed in the highest number of actors, recruiting them to adopt and spread these surgeons' surgical techniques.

There are key concealed actors, however, who were recruited before anyone else and who make any surgeon's knowledge possible: the patient or patients on whom these innovations are first tested and on whom a surgeon builds his or her case about surgical success. During the live demonstrations carried out during conferences, patients are already under anesthesia by the time they appear on camera, and they are regarded as passive objects of clinical study by the surgeons witnessing the surgery. The audience, therefore, is twice removed from the patients, whose welfare is entrusted to the surgeon. A Brazilian plastic surgeon I interviewed at the annual meeting of the Brazilian Society of Plastic Surgery, Dr. Marcio, assured me that these patients received a fair deal, since their surgeries were usually low cost or free of charge. Most of these patients were recruited in publicly funded hospitals and did not have the money to afford surgery in a private clinic. Dr. Marcio admitted that since the 1960s, when Ivo Pitanguy first made surgery available to the poor, Brazilian surgeons have had incomparable "access to a great number of patients for clinical trials, for educating new surgeons, as well as for research regarding one surgery or another." He firmly believed, however, that the social benefit outweighed any risks these patients undertook.

An American plastic surgeon I interviewed at the same conference had a more cynical take on it: "Brazilian surgeons are pioneers. They always have been. Our techniques we borrow and develop from their techniques. You know why? Because here they don't have the institutional and legal barriers to generat[ing] these new techniques. They can be as creative as they want to be. In the U.S. that is not the case: you always have the regulations, the FDA, on your back." The American surgeon believed that it was the lack of regulations and other legal red tape that allowed Brazilians plastic surgeons to be innovative, and he felt American regulations were *too* concerned with the safety of patients, thus preventing the creativity of surgeons to flourish. For both Dr. Marcio and the American surgeon, innovation was a good in itself—a sign of medical progress that guarantees Brazilian plastic surgery a prestigious place in knowledge production. A successful experimental setting, in other words, requires both regulatory flexibility and the unfettered access to bodies on which new, unproven techniques can be developed.

Generally, medical conferences merely provide doctors with information about the latest techniques; only rarely do they provide hands-on experience in how to carry out new medical procedures. A young German plastic surgeon I interviewed at a teaching hospital explained to me that he came to Brazil on a fellowship to complement the education he had gotten back home. He spent a few years in Germany learning reconstructive techniques such as burn grafts, but he felt his training in aesthetic surgery was lacking and knew that Brazil could provide this invaluable training as a result of the Pitanguy model of education. This German surgeon chose the most common route to learning aesthetic surgery in Brazil, which was to join an accredited plastic surgery course at a teaching hospital. Other options regularly used by doctors from other specialties consist of getting a degree in aesthetic medicine at a local teaching hospital, which takes less time than getting a plastic surgery degree, or informally learning how to perform plastic surgeries within the public health-care system. In Brazil it has become common to hear of gastroenterologists performing tummy tucks, gynecologists carrying out vaginal rejuvenations, dermatologists executing face-lifts, and otolaryngologists providing nose jobs. As I argued in chapter 2, the permeable boundaries between private and public health allow doctors to easily practice medicine in both settings, transferring knowledge they acquire in one to the other.

There is no controversy within the medical system over using the patients of publicly funded hospitals as experimental subjects—they are understood as acceptable subjects of clinical study who, in exchange, receive low-cost or free surgeries. What is highly controversial is the entrance of doctors who do not specialize in plastic surgery into a restricted field of knowledge, creating a turf war between specialties. The Brazilian Society of Plastic Surgery has repeatedly denounced the invasion of their field by doctors from other specialties, and it has attempted to legally limit the ability of such surgeons to perform plastic surgeries. The Brazilian legal system, however, has so far protected the right of doctors to perform all types of surgeries.[4] Plastic surgeons claim that while they have years of medical training at teaching hospitals and therefore represent less risk to patients, other doctors obtain "worthless" degrees in aesthetic medicine or acquire their skills haphazardly. The Brazilian Society of Aesthetic Medicine, which comprises a collection of doctors from a wide array of medical specialties, has countered that their field has international recognition and relies more on advanced technologies that are minimally invasive and thus safer.

The legal wrangling and public competition between these medical associations, however, conceal the ways in which both accredited teaching hospitals and nonaccredited forms of training externalize risk and transfer it to the bodies of low-income patients. Ivo Pitanguy's plastic surgery service for the poor at the Santa Casa da Misericórdia, for example, is located only a few blocks from a very similar service for low-income patients run by the Brazilian Society of Aesthetic Medicine.

Both are strategically located in the center of Rio de Janeiro and, thus, easily accessible to the working-class patients who come looking for a variety of medical practices that promise them beauty. Both also double as medical schools for doctors seeking to specialize either in plastic surgery or in aesthetic medicine. The discourse put forward by both medical schools is that they provide a humanitarian service that gives beauty to the unfortunate individuals who are deprived of it, and that they promote social inclusion through surgery.

As the director of the residency program in aesthetic medicine explained to me: "No one is a guinea pig here. [We] provide for the well-being of the population, help with their self-esteem, and promote their inclusion in society. . . . Appearance is one of the preponderant factors for individual success. Patients arrive with a lowly physiognomy, but leave with another perspective, exhibiting radical changes." In this discourse, the appearance of the patients defines their social worth: their poverty and suffering is epitomized by their "lowly physiognomy," while beautification is portrayed as a source of upward mobility and success. It is practically identical to the eugenics-inspired narrative used by Ivo Pitanguy to justify opening a plastic surgery service for the poor, which portrayed doctors as providing happiness and well-being to a population in dire need. The very infrastructure of plastic surgery in teaching hospitals depends on this biopolitical rationalization of beautification as being able to uplift not only individuals but also Brazil's poor population as a whole. Framing plastic surgery as a benevolent gift gains state and public support for surgeons' efforts, and the state always resolves any risk-benefit calculations in favor of the surgeons.

To give a concrete example, in late 2015 former president Dilma Rousseff approved new legislation that would provide free plastic surgery in publicly funded hospitals to women who have been subject to domestic violence. The logic of this legislation was that "by offering reconstructive surgery, the State collaborates to allow a woman to reconstitute herself as a citizen after suffering due to violence."[5] Not only is this service a problematic way to address the elevated rates of domestic violence in Brazil—it is a cosmetic solution that does nothing to prevent further violence or to address gender inequality—but it is also presented as a remedial form of justice, not as a form of medicalization that could itself cause additional harm to female bodies. These women are expected to assume any risks involved in the surgeries, and the benefits for the surgeons who will operate on these women and learn from their bodies are rendered invisible.

I am particularly struck by the notion that plastic surgery could help women reconstitute themselves as citizens, because, as Emilia Sanabria illustrates in her work on contraceptives, the term *citizenship* is strategically used in Brazilian public hospitals to discipline patients to submit their bodies to medical treatments and thereby become good citizens. Citizenship, in this context, becomes a biopolitical operation that differentiates the low-income patients who need to be managed by the state from the consumer-citizens who have access to private health care and thus have the privilege of taking responsibility for their own health.[6] I agree with Sanabria that authors like Nikolas Rose put too much emphasis on "active biological citizens" who lobby the medical community and the state for recognition of their own medicalized subjectivities, and who transform biopower into an individualized project of self-government.[7] It seems to portray all patients as having complete agency over their medical choices, and it misses the ways in which such projects of self-government are simply illusory for the poor. I also share the concern expressed by Deborah Heath, Rayna Rapp, and Karen-Sue Taussig that these definitions of selfhood through biology, despite giving rise to new forms of democratic participation, also have the potential to rekindle eugenic thinking by classifying certain biological characteristics as undesirable.[8] Nikolas Rose dismisses these concerns as anachronistic,[9] but he never considers experimental settings where patients are regarded not as consumers with rights but as targets of uplift in the name of national progress.

I use the term *cosmetic citizenship* to point out the contradictory aspects of submitting one's body to plastic surgery, where the aspirational aspects of gaining access to citizenship through beauty are tempered by one's becoming enmeshed in experimental settings that reduce one's autonomy. Here, I subscribe to Amy Brandzel's insight that citizenship is always a normative operation, one which "regulates and disciplines the social body in order to produce model identities," simultaneously promising inclusion while reproducing exclusionary structures.[10] Cosmetic citizenship exists because it offers affective promises regarding beauty, but it does not always deliver well-being or happiness. Cosmetic citizens are not deluded about the contradictions inherent in becoming experimental subjects. As one interviewee put it, "In return for our surgery, we are guinea pigs for the [medical] students, who already have the theory but still need the practice." Cosmetic citizens, however, inevitably compare this medical risk to the daily risks they suffer due to Brazil's entrenched inequalities.

For instance, some patients regard plastic surgery as innocuous in comparison to the larger context of urban violence and government neglect that has become common in Brazil, particularly in working-class neighborhoods. I had an extended conversation with the owner of a small beauty salon in the working-class neighborhood of Meriti, in Rio de Janeiro, who dismissed my questions about the risks of surgery with a wave of her hand and told me that beauty was something essential and worth any risk. She said that in neighborhoods like the one she lived in, "living itself is a risk—one could be mugged any day, anywhere, just walking down the street." Other women present in the salon told me that plastic surgeons were at least more trustworthy than the corrupt politicians and the inept government institutions who gave nothing in return for the trust that people put in them. In a context of precarity and inequity, the experimental settings of plastic surgery seem like a sensible risk to become entangled in, for a chance at beauty.

What happens when something goes wrong and the results of surgery are unsatisfactory or directly affect a patient's health? The media notices a case of medical malpractice only when it concerns a celebrity or when it leads to someone's death, and then blame is quickly assigned to the individual surgeon and his or her lack of experience, rather than to the medical system that has allowed plastic surgeries to proliferate. I talked to a medical-malpractice lawyer who explained to me that she had stopped taking cases related to plastic surgery, because the legal system in Brazil makes it very difficult to prove beyond a reasonable doubt that the plastic surgeon made an error and harmed the patient. It is relatively easy for surgeons to claim that the patient's suffering is the result of common medical complications that were not under their control.

The plastic surgeries performed on low-income patients, in particular, are much harder to prosecute as cases of malpractice, because they are labeled as reconstructive surgeries in order to justify them in the eyes of the state. While in the case of aesthetic surgeries, prosecutors are required to prove only that the negative outcome has harmed a patient "morally"—that is, that the patient suffered social and psychological harm owing to the surgery—in the case of reconstructive surgeries the prosecutor has to prove that the method used by the surgeon was inadequate and that it impaired the patient's health. Otherwise, the surgeon can claim that the health benefits of the reconstructive surgery, which is meant to improve bodily function rather than bodily aesthetics, outweighed the risks of a negative aesthetic outcome. Thus, a low-income patient who underwent plastic surgery in the public health-care system would first have to demonstrate that the surgery was mislabeled as reconstructive before being able to prosecute a doctor, something almost impossible to do without a paper trail to prove it. As I demonstrated in chapter 2, the agreement between a plastic surgeon and a patient to rename a particular aesthetic surgery as a reconstructive surgery happens only informally, as a special favor the doctor is doing for the patient, and it is never recorded on the forms submitted to the hospital or to the government.

The Brazilian Society of Plastic Surgery is alarmed about the escalating number of cases of medical malpractice that go to court, but it is mostly concerned with protecting its own members. In 2007, the SBCP dedicated a whole special issue of their official magazine, *Plastiko's*, to the legal responsibilities of plastic surgeons, providing them advice on how to defend themselves from accusations of malpractice. An article by SBCP's judicial consultant makes very clear that reconstructive surgeries are much less likely to be prosecuted by the justice system, because they are considered cures for existing ailments, and that only surgeries with purely aesthetic aims can lead to large awards for damages in favor of the patient. He gives as an example a woman who got a breast reduction surgery and ended up with asymmetrical breasts. Because her surgery was considered reconstructive, the judicial system ruled against her.[11] This issue of *Plastiko's* also recommended that surgeons get their patients to sign consent forms listing all the possible risks and complications the patient is assuming by undergoing surgery, which gives the doctor a certain amount of protection under the law. In the worst-case scenario, where a patient dies and it is proven that the surgeon was at fault, the average award for damages is two hundred thousand reais (about sixty thousand U.S. dollars)[12]—a paltry amount given the years of litigation and the exorbitant legal fees that pursuing compensation requires.

Ultimately, the magazine lays most of the blame for the rising number of cases of malpractice on doctors from other medical specialties invading the field of plastic surgery, and reminds SBCP members that the judiciary depends on the expert medical evaluations of specific plastic surgeons to determine whether a particular doctor caused a patient harm. These expert witnesses, one plastic surgeon argues, "are of enormous importance in the judicial process, and become the 'eyes of the judge' in all technical questions, executing the force of the law and the state."[13] In other words, plastic surgeons who are members of the SBCP evaluate the medical merits of a particular case, and they are predisposed to see doctors of other disciplines as unqualified to do aesthetic surgeries. I heard similar criticism at a meeting of the Brazilian Society of Aesthetic Medicine, where several doctors from other medical specialties complained that in cases of malpractice, the system is biased and is much more likely to give harsher sentences to doctors from other specialties than to plastic surgeons.

Cosmetic citizens are the weakest link in this assemblage of legal and medical responsibility, taking the fall whenever they suffer medical complications from plastic surgery. The rationality of plastic surgery makes it almost impossible for working-class patients to sue plastic surgeons who have harmed them, and thus they are asked to assume all responsibility stemming from risky experimental procedures carried out mostly by medical residents still in training. As James Holston has pointed out, citizenship has traditionally been used in Brazil to apply the law unequally and, thus, to differentiate citizens in entrenched hierarchical patterns. To be a "common citizen" is to be someone insignificant in Brazilian society and, thus, subservient to state power, in contrast to a person of importance who is considered above the law.[14] It is not surprising, therefore, that plastic surgeons and other doctors, as members of the elite, would seek to protect themselves from legal or medical prosecution in relation to patients they consider to be charity cases, on whom they are bestowing the gift of plastic surgery. Media outlets that blame victims of medical malpractice for their own "bad choices" reassert a logic of neoliberal responsibility that does not account for the ways in which patients are stripped of their autonomy as they become enmeshed in experimental settings as medical subjects. Cosmetic citizenship is incredibly alluring because many patients navigate its perilous waters and emerge unscathed, but it is also exceedingly unforgiving to those who suffer what Paul Farmer would call the "structural violence" of its logic.[15]

THE PROBLEM OF CONSENT

I met Celine, a woman in her late twenties, at a philanthropic teaching hospital in Belo Horizonte, where she was about to undergo a second plastic surgery. The first surgery, she told me, was carried out by a young plastic surgeon in another teaching hospital who had not yet completed his training, and who had promised to provide her a tummy tuck at no cost, paid for by the Brazilian universal health-care system. All Celine had to do was declare that she was suffering from a hernia and complain of unrelenting pain and intestinal problems. This would permit the surgeon to conduct major surgery, which he would call a hernia correction while actually performing a mini-abdominoplasty, a new technique that he claimed was not as invasive as a full abdominoplasty. Celine agreed, hopeful that she would get rid of the excess belly tissue that had bothered her since her second pregnancy.

When she awoke from the surgery, however, she found that her belly was deformed and uneven, with a scar much worse than the one left by a C-section, even though the surgeon had promised it would be similarly subtle. The young plastic surgeon offered to do a corrective surgery for Celine, again at no cost to her, but she refused, afraid he simply did not have enough experience to do a good job. It was not worth it, she told me, to denounce the doctor, or to try to sue him in court, because she would most likely get nothing out of it, and lawyers were too expensive. Instead, she decided to come to this philanthropic teaching hospital, where surgeries were not free but were low cost, and where she hoped she would find better, more skilled surgeons. Only by paying money, she told me, did you get a decent doctor, and only the wealthy got the best plastic surgeons available. This second surgery would represent a lot of money for her, but it was very important for her to try to recover a semblance of the body she once had. Corrective, secondary surgeries like this one are very common at this and other publicly funded hospitals—almost always related to unskilled surgeons who promised more than they could deliver.

Ana Maria was luckier. She told me about her hernia surgery, which had almost become a tummy tuck, while we were having some coffee and cake at her humble home on the periphery of Rio de Janeiro. She had worked as a maid for wealthier families for several decades before retiring recently, and now she mostly stayed at home, taking care of her ailing husband, who suffered from dementia. She was in excellent health, except for a recurring hernia problem that had become more and more painful as time went on. She went to see a doctor at the local free health clinic, who referred her to a gastrointestinal surgeon at a public hospital. This surgeon was very eager, she recollected, to perform the surgery to correct her hernia, but he strongly suggested she take the opportunity to get an abdominoplasty as well. Both surgeries, he guaranteed, would be covered by the universal health-care system and would not cost her a dime.

Ana Maria had her doubts, because this surgeon had not specialized in plastic surgery, and she understood that a tummy tuck was a surgery with additional risks, much more complex than her hernia correction. She suspected that the surgeon must have an additional motive for carrying out this surgery—what was in it for him? She reluctantly agreed, because her belly fat bothered her somewhat and the surgeon had made it sound like this plastic surgery would be an added benefit, something that would restore her youth. She checked into the hospital the morning of her two surgeries, only to discover that the anesthesiologist had vetoed the tummy tuck, refusing to put a woman of advanced age like Ana Maria under general anesthesia for any period of time longer than was absolutely necessary. The anesthesiologist accused the surgeon of wanting to learn how to do tummy tucks in order to carry them out in his private practice. "Just imagine," Ana Maria told me, "they almost cut me open like a pig to take out the fat!" Both she and Celine became experimental subjects on whom surgeons wanted to hone their skills in different techniques of abdominoplasty, justifying these surgeries as hernia corrections in the eyes of the state. Both patients were kept in the dark about the risks, and Ana Maria had not even actively sought plastic surgery—her hernia was a real health problem that a doctor took advantage of in his quest for knowledge.

Ana Maria's comment regarding being cut open like a pig reminds us of the fleshy messiness of surgery—the ways in which the scalpel is merely a refined kitchen knife that interacts with a flesh that resists being cut, and which bleeds after the scalpel goes in. As Tim Ingold argues, "The skin is not an impermeable boundary but a permeable zone of intermingling and admixture"—a living material that reminds us that every organism is always already entangled with the world around it.[16] Witnessing tummy tucks was a mesmerizing yet gruesome experience because the surgery consists in removing a wide section of skin and fatty tissue around a person's navel, stretching the skin to tighten the abdominal wall, and then, peculiarly, creating a new hole for the navel. The "excess" skin and fat are simply set aside to be discarded (fig. 12).

The body is not a passive object on which the surgery is performed but living matter that immediately reacts to the physical trauma it is undergoing, bleeding during the surgery and creating scar tissue during the healing process. Surgeons use several techniques to keep the patient from bleeding out, to prevent infection, and to suture the wounds they have created in a way that minimizes the resulting scar. An inexperienced surgeon, like the one who operated on Celine, risks causing irreparable harm to the body he is cutting into and then suturing—he can cut a vital artery, puncture a vital organ, fail to cauterize the wound, or misjudge how the patient's unique biology is reacting to his cuts and sutures.

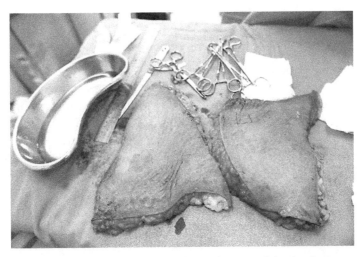

FIG 12. Tissue cut from a patient's abdomen during an abdominoplasty.
Photo courtesy of Vincent Rosenblatt.

I never saw a patient die on the operating table, but I witnessed many young surgeons struggling with the fact that a living, agential body on the operating table does not quite resemble the inanimate models they learned about in anatomy textbooks. When they are suturing the body in the final stages of the surgery, they suddenly realize that the cuts they have made on the body now render the flesh they are working on uneven, and that their patient's body will be inevitably misshapen or the scar too wide. A good surgeon is one who lets go of abstract models and learns to respond to a patient's body in real time, reading the signs of how a body is reacting to surgery. Brazilian medical schools pride themselves on providing their medical residents so much practice that, by the end of their residency, these surgical skills have become habitual and, hopefully, these doctors can now confront any eventuality that arises in their private practice.

Nonetheless, no medical resident has these skills at the beginning of his or her residency in a publicly funded hospital, and the risks of surgery are to a large extent inevitable, no matter how good a surgeon is or how much he has already learned. Additionally, I noticed a conflict between reducing risk for the patient and producing a better result. A particular surgery I witnessed at a teaching hospital in Belo Horizonte illustrates this. A medical resident called Felipe was carrying out one of his first liposuctions, and he was sweating heavily as he repeatedly inserted the cannula into the patient's abdomen and thighs. A cannula is a long cylindrical tool with holes in one end and a hose attached to a vacuum at the other end, which sucks the fat from the body and deposits it in a separate container. This fat, however, is not loose material floating in the body but tissue attached to skin and muscle, and thus it resists being removed.

Dr. Paulo, the chief surgeon at this medical school, came into the room occasionally to check on Felipe's progress, and kept insisting that Felipe was being too careful and was failing to remove important fat deposits. Felipe was afraid of doing something wrong that would risk the patient's health, such as puncturing a vital organ with the cannula or producing internal bleeding that could lead to an embolism. Dr. Paulo carefully managed Felipe's fears, however, by telling him that his future patients would be unhappy if the surgical result was negligible because not enough fat was removed. Felipe complied and applied even more force to the cannula. After the surgery was completed, however, he continued to worry, and so he monitored the patient frequently to make sure she was making good progress.

The patient in question was an elementary school teacher called Marly, who told me she was thrilled to have received a free liposuction from Dr. Paulo's team, despite the bruises that covered her body and the pain she was feeling. She told me she knew well that Dr. Paulo had a successful private practice in Rio de Janeiro, where he had only wealthy patients, and that he did not have to dedicate time to more modest patients like her to make money. Marly was comfortable with the fact that one of Dr. Paulo's medical residents would carry out the surgery, and that he would only supervise it, and she was also at ease with the idea that a publication might result from their study of her. She explained, "I know they are studying me, but I don't care. I wouldn't have a way to pay otherwise."

Learning from an experimental subject is not simply a question of applying technical knowledge to the body in an appropriate way. As Annemarie Mol reminds us, technical knowledge about the body does not come after practice, nor does it precede it—the technical and social versions of the body are intertwined and emerge simultaneously, even if they seem to contradict one another.[17] For medical residents who have only textbook knowledge of the body, the learning curve for a surgical procedure like liposuction is very high, but Dr. Paulo felt comfortable pushing his students because the experimental setting of the teaching hospital privileges a hands-on, practical knowledge that can push the boundaries of safety. In turn, this hands-on, risky approach also produces new technical knowledge about the body, because it leads to important publications by Dr. Paulo and his team.

Dr. Paulo was proud of the fact that he based his doctoral dissertation on new surgical techniques he had developed on these patients. He did not compete with doctors from other specialties but collaborated with them, particularly general surgeons who performed bariatric surgeries (also known as stomach-reduction surgeries) at this teaching hospital. He would help make the case that a given bariatric surgery was medically necessary even if the patient was not morbidly obese, in order for the public health-care system to cover it, and in return bariatric surgeons supplied him and his students with a constant flow of patients in need of postbariatric surgeries. The universal health-care system, he explained, barely paid him anything to carry out these surgeries, so he was in it for the challenge it represented and for the educational benefits it gave his students, more than for the money. By performing ten surgeries while developing a new technique, he already had enough data to publish a paper on the topic and present the results at plastic surgery conferences. Other doctors in Rio de Janeiro were envious, he claimed, of the access he had to these patients, as well as of the invaluable experience he was acquiring, making his weekly trips to Belo Horizonte very much worth it. His reputation had allowed him to open his own medical residency, which was a significant source of income and social capital.

Since Dr. Paulo had developed his dissertation while operating on these patients, he regarded it as perfectly fair for me to develop my anthropological research on these patients as well—and he largely disregarded my claims that I was more interested in the larger medical system that promoted plastic surgeries. As a result, it was common for him to ask his patients to disrobe in front of me, despite my evident discomfort. One of these patients, Dona Elza, insisted I could continue to interview her even after Dr. Paulo had asked her to remove her clothes completely so he could proceed to mark up her naked body and take several photographs of her (a typical procedure before surgery). She assured me that she was accustomed to this type of situation and had lost her shame. This was Dona Elza's second plastic surgery after a bariatric surgery that had allowed her to lose seventy-two kilograms. Her first surgery with Dr. Paulo had targeted her abdomen and was not entirely successful, because she had lost her navel to infection and had suffered a pulmonary embolism that nearly killed her. She was still thankful, however, to Dr. Paulo and one of his residents, who had been caring and sweet during her long recovery in the hospital.

When Dr. Paulo asked her if they could use her images for educational purposes, she calmly agreed and remarked with a laugh, "They can study me. I like to contribute something to the study of medicine. I am not a guinea pig; they call me their 'model.' . . . I'll come out in the *Playboy* of the medical school!" She also signed the consent form without reading it. Dona Elza's remark that she would "come out in the *Playboy* of the medical school" reveals the ways in which sexual innuendo softened the formality of the doctor-patient relationship. She was perhaps deploying humor to diffuse discomfort caused by the fact that she was nude in front of us and was agreeing to become an experimental subject. She did not know, at that point, if she would even survive that second surgery. As Donna Goldstein argues, sexually improper and even grotesque humor is very common in Brazil and seems to engage the absurdities of Brazilian inequality, simultaneously masking and revealing everyday forms of violence.[18] I would argue, however, that humor and the familiarity it represents also signal the ways in which the risks of surgery are offset through acts of affective intimacy on the part of both patient and doctor.

Dr. Paulo carefully managed his relationship with Dona Elza because she represented a valuable case study on which he was currently building new knowledge. I witnessed her second plastic surgery, a "circumferential flankplasty and cruroplasty" that removed skin from Elza's back in order to lift her buttocks, combining that procedure with liposuction, a surgery that Dr. Paulo admitted he and his residents were carrying out for the first time. He told me excitedly that this was a complex surgery that few people in Brazil or any other part of the world knew how to perform, and which confirmed his skill as a surgeon. His willingness to take this risk surprised me, given the complications Dona Elza had suffered after her previous surgery, but perhaps he was counting on the friendly relationship he and his residents had cultivated with her over the past few months in case anything went awry.

I saw Dona Elza again a few weeks later, when she came back for a checkup, which also allowed Dr. Paulo to take pictures of the surgical outcome. Dona Elza's surgery had been more successful this time around, and she was very happy with the result, telling me she felt younger and more attractive. She commented that her only pleasure before losing weight and getting these plastic surgeries had been to eat nonstop, and that now she felt she could "find pleasure in studying, working, and living life." Capitalizing on her mention of the word "pleasure," Dr. Paulo joked that she would also find newfound pleasure in having sex, and added that all the pictures he kept taking of her would turn her into the new Gisele Bündchen. His surgical skill, he said with a smirk, would allow her to wear those little bikinis that show off the buttocks. Dona Elza did not take offense at these sexually suggestive comments but laughed heartily along with him. It was common for Dr. Paulo to take these types of liberties with his low-income female patients, and he explained to me later that it was one of the ways he put patients at ease. He prided himself on producing compliant patients who came to him time and again for surgeries, and who put their trust in him despite any complications. He taught his medical residents techniques from neurolinguistics he had learned from a self-help book, and which he was convinced could persuade patients to accept all his suggestions, such as his recommendations for additional surgeries.

Despite all of Dr. Paulo's charm and confidence, however, he still had patients who were noncompliant. He complained to me once about a patient who refused to be part of an ongoing clinical study because her first surgery had caused an infection, which he considered to be a typical medical complication. He said the disadvantage of operating on low-income patients like this one was that they refused to follow proper procedure and did not get enough rest after surgery, returning to work too quickly, and that this led to undesirable results. He thus shifted the blame for undesirable results to his patients, ignoring the role played by his risky surgical techniques. Dr. Paulo also ignored the economic constraints that led many of the low-income patients I interviewed to carefully determine how many weeks they could afford to take off work before causing too much of a financial burden on their families. His main frame of reference was his wealthier patients, who could afford to not work for extended periods of time, and who had maids and personal nurses to help them during their convalescence.

I was never able to interview one of Dr. Paulo's noncompliant patients (he preselected patients for me to interview), but I did interview a hairdresser in her fifties called Karla, who had become a "model" for a plastic surgeon who promised her a face-lift. She would go to conferences with the surgeon, where he would perform live demonstrations and inject her face with an experimental "filler" that was supposed to temporarily rejuvenate her, all with the purpose of selling that product to other surgeons. She complied with this surgeon's demands for months but eventually tired of his broken promises regarding her face-lift, since he kept postponing it. Karla still admired the plastic surgeon for his skill but believed that he took advantage of her sincere desire for surgery.

I was struck by how she described her experience as a breach of trust—similar to how Renata and Celine described their experience as experimental subjects. All three women had placed their faith in doctors promising them beauty because they trusted the excellent reputation of Brazilian plastic surgery, and thus they expected a fair return for becoming an experimental subject. They were lashed in affectively before they even set foot in a hospital or medical office, but it was their trust in a particular surgeon or medical service that usually clinch the deal for them. Several patients mentioned that it was the lineage that a particular doctor or service could trace to Ivo Pitanguy that put them at ease.

Most of the literature on experimental subjects in medical settings has overlooked the importance of affect in engendering consent, putting emphasis instead on the structural inequalities that influence patients' decisions. Adriana Petryna, for example, describes how pharmaceutical companies and their contractors conduct clinical trials in developing nations because it gives them access to large populations of patients who are economically vulnerable and who perceive clinical trials as a way to get access to new medical developments usually denied to them. This allows regulatory agencies to transfer all responsibility to the market and to individual "biological citizens" who are supposed to manage their own health and be aware of the risks they are taking.[19] In Petryna's earlier work on Chernobyl, however, we get a clear sense that biological citizens' relationship to medical regimes is always permeated by emotional claims of self and belonging.[20]

Similarly, Lawrence Cohen asks us to consider the fact that organ sellers in India are too concerned with paying off their crushing debt to consider the long-term effects of selling a kidney to a wealthy recipient.[21] Cohen remarks on the presumed "operability" of these patients—the ways in which they have negotiated their belonging within the state through "invasive medical commitments"—but he only hints at the ways these commitments depend on intimacy and other affective attachments.[22]

Roberto Abadie comes the closest to considering affect in his study of professional guinea pigs in Philadelphia, where he describes risk perception as situated in the affective and interpersonal elements of social relationships, which ground the choices that trial participants make in their immediate experiences rather than in any knowledge of risks detailed in the consent forms they sign.[23] I think Cohen, Petryna, and Abadie are right to point out how universalist applications of consent erase the complex realities and contingencies that shape patients' difficult choices, but these authors do not account for the ways in which consent is interwoven with powerful forms of affect, such as hope for a better future, trust in the medical system, and transitory intimacy in doctor-patient relationships.

When we account for affect contained in consent, we come to realize why patients' decisions would not become more "rational" with additional information about the risks they are taking. It is not simply the case that structural inequalities cloud the judgment of experimental subjects, or that they simply limit these subjects' options. Structural inequalities shape the very way that medical regimes *feel* and create the conditions in which any semblance of decision-making can emerge. Dona Elza signed her consent form without reading it because she knew perfectly well that the document provided no reliable information and that her health was now in the hands of others—she relied instead on an intuitive feeling that she could trust the surgeons who wanted to study her body to gain knowledge.

Intuition, as Brian Massumi argues, is not the opposite of rationality but, rather, is a rational operation "performed nonreflectively, [while you are] absorbed in the immediacy of perception's emergence. . . . [You are] following what you viscerally feel to be the best course. . . . [By following your intuition] you have performed an *embodied thinking-feeling*." Massumi provides the example of a person suddenly confronted with a bull in a field to illustrate how this embodied form of cognition can produce immediate, bodily reactions—a type of rationality that does not go through the assessments and calculations that one would expect.[24] Perhaps we should think of vulnerable patients as living in a state of precariousness that demands they act intuitively, thinking-feeling through the limited choices they are given. All rational choice is illusory, because it denies the ways that all social actors are always already entangled with the world around them; but the illusion becomes more evident when we talk about experimental subjects whose bodies have been made "bioavailable" for the production of medical knowledge.[25] Their embodied decisions allow us to notice the ways in which they are not simply docile in response to power, but agential actors in their own right, affectively engaging with the world around them.

THE SOCIAL LIFE OF IMPLANTS

Although plastic surgeons are not in the same vulnerable position as the experimental subjects they rely on, it would be problematic to represent them as more rational or calculating than their patients. Annemarie Mol points out that neither patients nor doctors "master the realities enacted out there, but . . . are involved in them. There are, therefore, no independent actors standing outside reality, so to speak, who can choose for or against it."[26] In other words, when we consider the choices that surgeons make, we must denaturalize the tendency to portray them as masters of their own domain who manipulate patients into compliance. The reality is that plastic surgeons, too, are seduced by the biopolitical regimes they promote, and they become affectively invested in the rationalities of their practice, no matter the cost.

For an ethnographer, it is hard to investigate the decision-making process of plastic surgeons, because in ordinary circumstances their medical knowledge has acquired a taken-for-granted quality and is not questioned by any of the participating actors. Bruno Latour describes these indisputable scientific facts as having become "black boxed," and he suggests that we follow the controversies that are still open and in dispute to examine how scientists settle competing claims and produce knowledge.[27] One such controversy is the one surrounding one of the most renowned but contentious plastic surgery techniques that has come out of Brazil, known as *bioplastia,* or "bioplasty." I do not claim that bioplasty is riskier than the average plastic surgery—liposuction has a much higher mortality rate, for example[28]—but bioplasty is an interesting case study because it became widely controversial during the time when I was carrying out fieldwork. While some surgeons claimed it was a highly experimental technique with little evidence to prove its safety, other surgeons defended it as a groundbreaking form of surgical enhancement that was a game changer in the industry. As Lesley Sharp argues, highly experimental medical practices provide ethnographers with great insights into the "moral thinking" that scientists use to justify controversial practices.[29] I find that the controversy over bioplasty particularly reveals plastic surgeons' beliefs about the plasticity of race and class in the Brazilian body politic, and it demonstrates how they understand their role in improving the population.

As a technique, bioplasty consists of a liquid compound called polymethyl methacrylate (PMMA), known in English as acrylic glass or plexiglass, which is injected directly into the muscular tissue of the face or body in order to permanently reshape this tissue. Its advocates claim that PMMA is highly "biocompatible," meaning the human body commonly shows no adverse reactions to the compound, and that the proof of this lies in the fact that the compound has been used safely for decades in dentures, in intraocular lenses placed by ophthalmologists, and as bone cement in orthopedic surgery. Its use in aesthetic procedures, however, is a relatively recent Brazilian innovation.

Doctors call PMMA a liquid implant, in the sense that it is meant to replace other types of injections as well as solid silicone implants, thus providing patients with a cheaper and easier way to alter their bodies and eliminating the need to go to a hospital. An estimated sixty liters (approximately fifteen gallons) of PMMA is used every month for aesthetic procedures in Rio de Janeiro alone.[30] At about two hundred dollars per application of a few milliliters, bioplasty produces millions of dollars in profit every year for the laboratories that produce the compound. Today, it is one of the most widespread and profitable aesthetic treatments in Brazil.

The success of bioplasty is clearly linked to the claim that it can instantaneously reshape a person's features and make a pliable body conform to normative beauty standards. The promise of limitless modification—frequently touted in advertisements for bioplasty—is so alluring for both doctors and patients that it trumps the enormous medical risks associated with the technique. The Brazilian Federal Council of Medicine issued a warning about the technique in 2006, asking doctors to be aware that its long-term effects were unknown, and to inform patients that advertisements about bioplasty's ability to transform the body were "fantastic and exaggerated."[31] Despite the warning, the council allowed the practice of bioplasty to continue.

I first heard about bioplasty during a plastic surgery conference in Rio de Janeiro, where a renowned plastic surgeon gave a talk about an extensive reconstructive surgery he had performed on a patient who lost half of her nose and right cheek to necrosis after a dermatological application of bioplasty. The patient had undergone bioplasty applications ten years earlier with no complications, but this time she suffered an intense immuno-allergic reaction that led to a large loss of tissue. She required several surgeries to correct the damage and was nonetheless left with an extensive scar on her face. The surgeon, genuinely puzzled about this turn of events, asked the audience, "Bioplasty was a consecrated technique; what happened here?"

When I interviewed this surgeon at length, he confirmed that there had been several dozen similar cases of patients suffering necrosis after applications of PMMA (see fig. 13 for one such example), but the question remained whether the error is in the product itself or in the person who applies it. As a member of the Federal Council of Medicine, the surgeon was part of the regulatory board that determined which medical

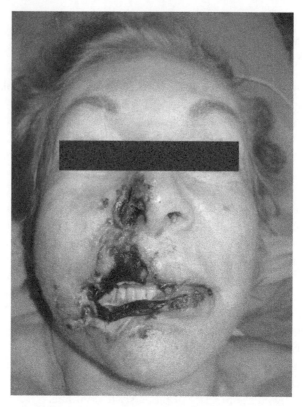

FIG 13. Extensive necrosis in a patient after an application of polymethyl methacrylate. Photo courtesy of Anderson Castelo Branco.

procedures were safe to use on the public, but he was reluctant to forbid bioplasty. Given the great number of people who had undergone the procedure, he argued, condemning the technique could lead to widespread public commotion and an avalanche of lawsuits. The surgeon also said that despite his concern about the technique, he was against prohibiting it because of its important reconstructive applications for the treatment of lipodystrophy in HIV-positive patients.[32] A few months later, I heard the same surgeon recommend the technique to his students, calling it a "formidable tool" that does not yet have an equivalent in plastic surgery. He seemed to have completely dismissed as an exceptional occurrence the case of the woman he had treated for necrosis, which apparently did not warrant even a warning to his students about the possible risks of bioplasty.

Like other experimental techniques, bioplasty was first developed on the bodies of low-income patients in public hospitals, but it became available for use on the general public without a proven track record of safety. In other words, the imaginary of bioplasty as a "formidable tool" trumped the need for a guarantee of safety, which normally would be required before a technique can be transferred from public hospitals to private clinics. There is controversy over who invented bioplasty, because a surgeon from Rio de Janeiro claims that he and his medical students first tested the aesthetic use of PMMA in a public hospital, perceiving its potential. He told me that the surgeon who today is known as the inventor won all the plaudits only because he was the first to gain official approval to produce the compound for medical use under a trademarked name.

As Bruno Latour argues, controversies over the authorship of a particular scientific development reveal the underlying networks that built support for its eventual success.[33] The laboratory that trademarked PMMA under the name *bioplasty* had a head start over other laboratories, and its advertisements for the product made the claim that bioplasty could replace many of the more invasive plastic surgeries, representing a new way of modifying the body without cutting into it. This not only provided the illusion of safety but was also a smart way to market this product across the aisle to doctors other than plastic surgeons. Bioplasty, for example, has been hugely successful among dermatologists and doctors specializing in aesthetic medicine, because it requires little training in comparison to other aesthetic procedures and seems to promise more in return. Other laboratories also went on to market applications of PMMA, but under different names, which have not captured the imagination of doctors or users in the same way. There is something about the name *bioplasty* that communicates very clearly the aim of the product, because it emphasizes the plasticity of biology, and because the suffix -*plasty* connects this aesthetic procedure to other forms of recognized plastic surgery, such as rhinoplasty.

I do not, however, want to reduce bioplasty's success to simply the strength of certain marketing techniques, to the power of its laboratories, or to the number of allies that it has recruited outside of plastic surgery. According to Emily Martin, anthropologists should be suspicious of Latour's claim that the scientific advances that triumph are simply those able to build the strongest networks or lash in the largest number of allies, accumulating the most actors and laboratories in their favor. This account portrays scientists as rational economic actors solely focused on enrolling the support of others, like capitalists accumulating knowledge-production instead of money.[34] What fascinates me about bioplasty is its resilience despite scandal, as well as the way doctors rush to defend the practice in the face of frightening results—there is something happening here that defies our notion of medical science as composed of rational economic actors who carefully calculate the costs and benefits of a particular technique.

For example, in April 2007, the influential television program *Fantástico,* which airs Sunday evenings on the Globo Network, covered the case of a woman who went blind in one eye shortly after applications of bioplasty near her periorbital area. Her doctor denied that the bioplasty had caused it, and insisted she must have had a preexisting condition that affected her eyes. The television program also talked about a study with rats conducted by the University of Brasilia, which determined that PMMA is a dangerous compound that can migrate to the kidneys and liver and cause health problems. The journalists covering the topic unequivocally condemned bioplasty as a dangerous technique and warned patients to be wary of doctors advertising it. After the program aired, a few of the surgeons I interviewed became a little more hesitant about defending bioplasty, but most kept insisting it was a valid technique and that the television program had been biased and inaccurate. Their attachment to the technique superseded their need to protect their reputation as guardians of their patients' safety.

The next year, in June 2008, the Fifth Global Conference on Aesthetic Medicine, which took place in Rio de Janeiro, featured two panels and a keynote lecture dedicated solely to defending bioplasty. In front of their peers, doctors from several disciplines took a stand against the mounting critiques of bioplasty and claimed that there were more than a hundred studies proving its safety and more than a million satisfied patients to date. Some of these doctors admitted that they worked as consultants in the laboratories that produce PMMA, but others said they were simply converts who believed wholeheartedly in bioplasty.

Occasional complications, these panelists argued, are inherent in any medical treatment. One doctor claimed that the "concerted campaign to tarnish the product" was a consequence of the threat bioplasty represents to conventional plastic surgeons who are unwilling to admit their techniques are outdated. Presenters passionately argued that, despite any risks, to turn one's back on bioplasty would be to renounce one of the most powerful advances in medical history. Injectable implants, a plastic surgeon claimed, were a "phenomenal weapon that aesthetic medicine possesses[,] . . . a dream of defeating all afflictions . . . [by] completely modifying bodily structures." Using bioplasty, another claimed, the surgeon is "transformed into a sculptor" who can "make the ugly beautiful[,] . . . transforming shadows into light and creating points that illuminate the face." The doctor's power to dispel darkness and ugliness from a patient's features was not simply rhetorical, however, but was confirmed by the before-and-after pictures documenting the transformations of patients. By altering the angles and proportions of the chin, cheekbones and nose, doctors explained, the face of the patient was made to resemble those of fashion models and other international beauty icons. The improvement of the patients was not a subjective evaluation but a measurable fact verified through anthropometry.

The hyperbolic language used to describe bioplasty, as well as the passion with which the technique was defended, indicates that this experimental technique resonates at a visceral level with the affective promises that attract doctors to beautification in the first place. The narrative about bioplasty relies on the audience's preestablished perception that only certain features are aesthetically desirable, and that the power to engineer those features on the human body—and on the body politic as a whole—can be interpreted only as medical progress. This biopolitical illusion is so powerful that doctors are surprisingly willing to choose controversial but revolutionary innovations, for which there are no guarantees of safety, over more conventional techniques with less potential.

The innovations that affectively capture the imagination of surgeons and spread quickly in hospitals, clinics, and consultation rooms are not only those that are most lucrative but also those that promise to produce the most impressive transformations in the Brazilian population. Bioplasty is seductive because it is always characterized as having an enormous potential to reshape bodily structures altogether, literally creating high cheekbones and square jawlines where there were none before. Doctors describe it as a powerful weapon they do not have the luxury to discard, and they prefer to believe in its safety despite the accumulating evidence against it. Thus, while Latour portrays all scientific controversies as teleologically headed toward closure in one direction or another, I found that plastic surgery and aesthetic medicine produce endless controversies that refuse closure altogether. Risky techniques like bioplasty, which have been controversial since their inception, are able to continuously recruit new allies at the same time that they gain new detractors, because they affectively lash in new actors who want to believe in the technique's biopolitical power.

Some doctors are more explicit than others about the future they envision for the nation through bioplasty. For example, a dermatologist on one of the bioplasty panels I mentioned earlier claimed that the facial characteristics of all patients could be grouped and managed according to the four different temperaments: phlegmatic, choleric, melancholic, and sanguine. He argued the last three should be enhanced, respecting the patient's temperament, and proceeded to explain in detail how bioplasty could bring out the best in each patient. In contrast, he warned his audience, the phlegmatic face should simply be eliminated, because it represents the "features of the poor, with a round face, drooping eyes, receding chin and general weakness. . . . [A]ssassins have this type of face, and our society has no place for it." Bioplasty, this doctor argued, could transform a phlegmatic face into a more pleasing sanguine face, one that was more elongated and presented stronger, more aquiline features.

In every other context, I heard the phrase "round face" being attributed to poor people from northeastern Brazil, and it was not surprising that the dermatologist attributed to them a criminality that he believed could be easily read on their features—Brazil has a long legacy of using Lombrosian criminology to stigmatize underprivileged groups.[35] What was unexpected was his claim that bioplasty should literally excise certain physical characteristics from the social body, associating beautification with a eugenic enterprise. Despite the claim that bioplasty gives more agency to the patient by allowing him or her to remain awake and provide the surgeon with feedback during the injections, surgeons have a fixed idea of which physical characteristics produce beauty and which produce ugliness. They also believe that bioplasty can rearrange facial structures completely, transforming Brazil's population into a more aesthetically pleasing body politic.

When I asked one of the main advocates of bioplasty, Dr. Adilson, why he thought bioplasty and similar beautification techniques were in such high demand in Brazil, he answered, "Miscegenation improved the *eugenia* [eugenesis] of the population, and beautification techniques aid eugenics because they help people remain youthful and improve themselves." I had not asked Dr. Adilson about race, miscegenation, or eugenics, but those racial questions were at the forefront of his approach to his medical discipline. He seemed to think that beautification was, at its core, a eugenic endeavor that complemented the work of miscegenation. Like other surgeons invested in a raciology of beauty, whom I described in the previous chapter, he imagined miscegenation as a force of constant innovation that produces hybrid racial subjects who, as a collective, slowly approximate a Brazilian ideal. Miscegenation, therefore, becomes a central engine of national identity, but it cannot accomplish that work alone.

Doctors who most closely associate their innovative beautification techniques with the engine of miscegenation can also portray their science as capable of improving the nation's population, complementing its aesthetic work. This is the key to why certain techniques that promise doctors the ability to alter and enhance physical features at will are perceived as the most revolutionary, and why doctors are so unwilling to part with them, despite the risks. This association between racial improvement and beautification sometimes becomes more explicit, but more often it occurs implicitly, below the level of awareness. One of the advertisements for bioplasty, for example, simply makes references to how the technique can produce the characteristics "found among the most beautiful *mulheres Ocidentais* [Western women]" and assumes the target audience will equate Western features with whiteness. The text is accompanied by before-and-after pictures of men and women who have been "redesigned" by bioplasty and have gained sharper and squarer features. Since the narrative states that the patients portrayed in the after pictures have attained typical Western beauty, the before pictures are racialized as non-Western.

These subtly racialized semiotic codes underwrite the drive behind certain innovations, like bioplasty, because surgeons become affectively attached to new techniques that supposedly increase the pliability of the body. Despite a growing number of studies that show that PMMA is a risky technique that can potentially cause nodules under the skin, can migrate to different tissues of the body, including the liver and kidneys, and can cause extremely adverse reactions like blindness and the necrosis of facial tissue,[36] there are enough doctors who remain advocates of the technique to foster its continued use and legitimacy. These doctors always dismiss adverse reactions to PMMA as caused by improper applications rather than admit the technique itself is inherently dangerous. Not only does this suggest that surgeons' preferences are not driven by rational choice, but it also implies that surgeons offer little resistance to becoming enmeshed in rationalities that they find intuitively superior to cost-benefit analysis. These intuitive rationalities are shaped by their own class and race privilege, and their embodied perceptions of what is beautiful and good.

The one actant that refuses to substantiate the claimed rationality of bioplasty is the human body itself, with its tendency to react adversely to PMMA injections. Here, I find Ingold's critique of Latourian actor-network theory useful, particularly his description of actants as having indeterminate boundaries, as not being discrete objects like in Latour's description. If the controversy over bioplasty refuses closure, it is because bodies "can exist and persist only because they *leak:* that is, because of the interchange of materials across ever-emergent surfaces."[37] Despite the biopolitical desire to produce bodies as discrete units of intervention, and despite the belief that PMMA is easily enfolded into human biology and allows surgeons to shape the body in predictable fashion, the very materiality of the body reveals a more complex experience of embodiment that is always in motion and which interacts with injectable implants in volatile ways—necrosis, rejection, absorption, nodulation, migration. If we think of the body as a relational material that is continuously emerging from its surroundings, it can never be lashed into the production of medical knowledge without severely simplifying its way of being in the world.

UNFULFILLED PROMISES

In the first chapter of this book, I described how neo-Lamarckian eugenicists imagined they would create a more beautiful nation by intervening in the population's access to health-care, providing them with basic sanitation and hygienic education. Toward the end of this book, we return to a vision of eugenics as beautification, but one that brandishes plastic surgery as the way to achieve that aim. I remember sitting with Dr. Paulo at Rio de Janeiro's bus station, waiting for the bus that would take us to Belo Horizonte, where I would get to see the surgeries he carried out on low-income patients. Dr. Paulo turned to me and, pointing to the people in the bus station, said,

> See these people? The *povão* [masses] who elect our corrupt politicians? Our country would not be the way it is, if it weren't for them. . . . Plastic surgery, however, is a force for good. I'm not simply a plastic surgeon; I'm someone who can rebuild people, I'm an instigator of happiness, I'm a catalyst for change. . . . I seek to teach my patients how to constantly improve themselves. Plastic surgery can generate a revolution in this country and change our very way of being. It is an extension of medicine, providing mental as well as physical health.

Dr. Paulo clearly understood his profession as much more than simply beautifying the people he worked on. He was very concerned about the direction the country was going, particularly under the rule of the leftist

Workers' Party, but believed that the aesthetic enhancements he provided to his low-income patients were part of a larger project of uplifting the poor and providing an aesthetic revolution in the nation.

As we have seen, this image of plastic surgeons as humanitarians is part of a biopolitical and legal rationality that soft-pedals the risks of surgery, externalizing the costs of surgery onto the bodies of patients. The experimental settings of plastic surgery promise citizenship through beauty but enmesh low-income patients in networks of knowledge production that render them into experimental subjects for clinical studies usually carried out by medical residents. Dr. Paulo's neoliberal logic in teaching patients how to "improve themselves" relied on an understanding of beauty as a rational choice. He did not perceive calculations of risk as relational and intuitive, and as arising from embodied perceptions that complicate our notions of autonomy. The tenet of rational choice cannot encompass a body that has agential capacities in its own right, and it ignores how the lived body is always moving, always emerging, and always entangled with its surroundings.

Nonetheless, it might be dangerous to put too much emphasis on the agential capacities of the body or to discount the ability of biopolitical rationalities to mobilize and act upon patients and their biologies. Dr. Paulo's hyperbolic description of his own medical discipline had very real effects on the experimental subjects of plastic surgery, as well as on the patients whose reconstructive surgeries are not considered profitable or useful by the existing medical system. At Dr. Paulo's medical school in Belo Horizonte, I was struck by how much two of his medical residents, Antonia and Felipe, hated to clean out bedsores, a type of skin ulcer that is common in people who are immobilized or confined to a bed for long periods of time. At this particular hospital, it was the responsibility of the plastic surgery team to surgically treat bedsores through a process known as debridement, which removes any dead tissue with a scalpel and is extremely painful. Dr. Paulo relegated this work to his residents, who constantly complained about it. Antonia once told me she wished a particular patient would simply die so she would not have to deal with her bedsores.

The patient in question was an old black woman who was clearly from a poor background. She was only skin and bones, had no teeth left, and seemed to have a serious developmental disability or psychological disorder, because she was unable to speak. No one seemed to know her name. I witnessed as Felipe held this woman down and Antonia proceeded to cut away the extensive necrotic tissue lining her bedsores, while the patient moaned and cried, obviously in severe pain. When the anesthesiologist present at the surgery asked if the patient should be anesthetized, Felipe responded that it was not worth it. There was a certain cruelty to their treatment of this patient, which dismissed her humanity in basic ways and contrasted sharply with the kind of care and attention that Dona Elza received to assure her compliance. Bedsores as egregious as these are already a symptom of neglect, since patients develop them only when they are abandoned on a bed or wheelchair for too long. As João Biehl argues, although Brazil's purported aim is to provide basic health care to all its citizens, the poorest of the poor are abandoned in overcrowded hospitals and infirmaries, where they live out a form of social death even before their human life is extinguished.[38]

There is no reason for plastic surgeons to affectively lash such destitute patients into their networks of care, since they are not useful to them. The question of who gets cared for in the Brazilian medical system, and what surgical interventions are valued, is central to any critique of plastic surgery. While the use of aesthetic plastic surgery continues to expand in Brazilian public hospitals, compelled by the need to train new surgeons and develop new techniques—and based on a rationality that sees beauty as central to national progress—the rest of the public health-care system suffers from a lack of economic and human resources. According to surveys of users of the public health-care system, the dearth of doctors is the main issue they face when attempting to get medical care.[39] For example, there is a severe shortage of pediatricians in several Brazilian states, which seems to be caused mainly by the fact that it is one of the worst remunerated medical disciplines in Brazil.[40] During my fieldwork, I noticed that medical residents specializing in other disciplines would openly express their desire to switch and specialize in plastic surgery instead, attracted by the potential income it would represent to them.

The recent economic crisis has probably put more pressure on medical residents to consider their eventual salary when deciding on their medical specialization. The crisis has also led Brazil's new neoliberal government to make sweeping cuts in the health-care system, putting in jeopardy primary care and the prevention campaigns for mosquito-transmitted diseases.[41] Only the municipality of Belo Horizonte has taken the step of cutting funding for elective surgeries to face this crisis, but it insisted that the cut was merely temporary,[42] and most other local governments prefer to make cuts in other areas with less symbolic capital. It will take a lot of political will to loosen the hold that plastic surgery has on the Brazilian public health-care system, and I do not see this occurring in the foreseeable future. Beauty, after all, has been established as a basic health right, and even patients who suffer the consequences of trusting in plastic surgeons still believe that the promise of beauty is the key to happiness.

Thinking of Beauty Transnationally

Nilse's previous face-lift surgery had left her with an uneven result on one side of her face. The doctor who operated on her agreed to give Nilse all her money back, to avoid a lawsuit, and she decided to reinvest the money in a second face-lift, this time at the Santa Casa. Unlike other patients who had suffered a setback, Nilse was still upbeat. She spoke very highly of Pitanguy, whom she described as "a global reference, a great surgeon," and Nilse was confident that his students would do a better job than her previous surgeon. Nilse, perhaps more than any other working-class patient I interviewed, seemed highly conscious of how Brazilian surgery and Brazilian women were perceived internationally: "Brazilians prioritize beauty even over health problems, because Brazilian women are seen as beautiful all over the world. We have a diverse beauty due to miscegenation, and we Brazilian women are seen as possessing a unique beauty. *Morenas* [brunettes] and *loiras* [blondes], *morenas* with blue eyes. . . . While Austrian and German women are blonde, and Colombian women are brunettes, we have both. We have a mixture, and no single beauty norm predominates, so every Brazilian has a different way of being beautiful."

While most other working-class patients told me personal stories of their struggles with becoming beautiful, Nilse told me a more abstract story about beauty's centrality in the transnational imaginary. In her view, Brazilian women care so much about beauty because they have a global reputation to live up to, and this reputation is clearly linked to

Brazil's imagined racial diversity. Nilse's light skin might explain her optimistic view that all types of racial backgrounds had a place in the imaginary of beauty, although she tellingly did not include black or indigenous women in her narrative of racial mixture, only *morenas* and *loiras* (although *morena* is an elastic term that can include people with brown skin). Yet she still felt the call to become beautiful in order to meet transnational expectations regarding Brazilian beauty, and she trusted Ivo Pitanguy because of his international reputation in the discipline of plastic surgery.

Nilse's comments reminded me of the way people in the United States frequently react to my research. Many Americans have commented that Brazilians, indeed, are the most beautiful people in the world—that Brazilians are known for plastic surgery, for supermodels like Gisele Bündchen and Adriana Lima, and for exposing their bodies at the beach or during Carnival. The images of Brazil that circulate globally are of scantily clad female bodies and the beauty work associated with them, and they produce a tropical touristic imaginary that then sells beautification practices like "the Brazilian bikini wax" and "the Brazilian butt lift" to women around the world.

Beauty is always transnational in scope, even as it is shaped by national imaginaries of racial mixture and by local gender relations and class struggles. In this book, I have turned to affect as well as biopolitics in order to provide a more complex account of beauty, one that explains it as a social relation that is not static but, rather, always in flux. The affective and biopolitical dimensions of beauty can also be useful in understanding it as a transnational practice, and can explain why beauty does not respect national boundaries but instead moves easily from one context to another, acquiring different lexicons and tones depending on the body politics it moves through. Using Arjun Appadurai's terminology, we can claim that beauty travels through specific circuits such as mediascapes (the transnational media representations of beauty and beauty practices), technoscapes (the international exchange of medical and nonmedical technologies to beautify the body), financescapes (the transnational financial power of the cosmetic, fashion, and beauty-pageant industries), ideoscapes (political and touristic imaginaries of beauty around the globe), and ethnoscapes (the global movement of models, plastic surgeons, and other beauty producers).[1] Appadurai's concept of global flows, however, does not explain why beauty moves in particular ways and what impels its movement, and this is where biopolitics and affect become particularly useful.

TRANSNATIONAL WAYS OF SEEING

My friend Priscila had many questions about my research on plastic surgery, but mainly she wanted to know how long the queues were in publicly funded hospitals, how safe the surgeries were, and what other low-cost options she had for obtaining liposuction. I had met Priscila in Rio while taking a folkloric dance course, and we quickly bonded over the beers we had after each class ended, partaking in what we jokingly called the "Club of the Big-Bellied Dancer." Priscila and I remained friends long after the dance course was over, because we shared the same sense of humor and our love of both dancing and good conversation.

Priscila was only slightly overweight, but she was very self-conscious about her figure and had tried everything under the sun to lose weight, including exercise, diet pills, and therapy, to no avail. She felt devalued by the men she dated, and complained how job opportunities were always limited because of her gender, her weight, and the color of her skin. Despite her two postgraduate degrees and ability to speak three languages, she was never offered anything above a clerical position in any company, and she saw others being promoted before her. Because of her humble background, she also lacked the connections necessary to make it in Rio de Janeiro's corporate world. Priscila's weight was a constant refrain in her emails—she told me several times her life would improve if she could simply lose some weight, because she imagined it would make her more of a catch in the marriage and job markets. Worried about her safety, I always tried to gently dissuade her from getting plastic surgery, and I shared some of the horror stories I had heard from patients whose surgeries had gone terribly wrong. Priscila went so far as to schedule liposuction with an inexpensive doctor from her working-class neighborhood, but she canceled it after one of that doctor's patients died during surgery.

Priscila's perspective about herself changed somewhat when she decided to join an international dating site, which put her in contact with mostly European men looking for relationships with Brazilian women. Suddenly, she began to receive flattering comments from men she found handsome (because they were blond and white) and who did not have any problem with the color of her skin or her weight, but found her particularly attractive and showered her with compliments. A couple of these men, one from Sweden and another from Norway, made the trip to Brazil to meet her and were surprisingly serious about their desire to have a long-term relationship with her. Priscila was hesitant about leaving her family in Brazil to pursue a relationship in a cold Nordic country, but she did visit Norway once and was amazed by how people reacted to her *brasilidade* (Brazilianness), as she called it—a combination of her bodily presence, her outgoingness, and her charm. She began to see herself in a different light, noticing she possessed a type of bodily capital she had not recognized and which was not merely aesthetic.

Priscila did not stop desiring plastic surgery, but she began to realize that her body was not the issue—what mattered was the way she looked at herself. In one of her emails after that trip, she wrote, "I used to focus all my anxiety on losing weight. Today, I do not focus on that anymore. Working, being healthy, having love for myself . . . those are my new priorities." I am not suggesting that Priscila's relationships with foreigners were redemptory in any way, because as Gregory Mitchell and Erica Lorraine Williams argue, working-class Brazilians' international sexual liaisons are permeated by ambiguous power relationships that complicate our notions of sexual economies and racial exoticism.[2] I am interested, however, in what happens to Brazilian beauty norms when they travel beyond national boundaries and are transformed by other ways of doing beauty. Priscila's trip to Norway opened her to new ways of seeing herself, even if how she was perceived there might have depended on globally circulating stereotypes of Brazilians. It was also merely a temporary respite from the real discrimination that she faced when she returned home to Brazil, but it allowed her to make beauty norms less of a priority in her life.

The transnational circulation of beauty, however, sometimes reinforces rigid notions of what is beautiful rather than opening up possibilities for rethinking beauty. I found this to be particularly true when Brazilian medical discourse traveled outside the nation's borders, carrying with it assumptions about racial improvement through surgery. For example, at a conference for alumni of Ivo Pitanguy's medical school, a plastic surgeon from Bolivia made a presentation on her surgical treatment of the "Andean nose," which she explained was an adaptation of the surgeries she had learned in Brazil to correct the "negroid nose." The surgeon claimed that the Andean nose was a typical physical feature of Bolivia's indigenous population and probably represented an evolutionary adaptation to the low oxygen levels at high altitudes, but that she and her Bolivian patients preferred noses that made them closer to the mestizo, mixed-race ideal. As an example of the Andean nose that required intervention, she used a photograph of the leftist president of Bolivia, Evo Morales, seemingly conflating his political program of defending indigeneity with an imagined ugliness.

In chapter 5, I made the argument that plastic surgeons' approach to the "negroid nose" is particularly revealing of the ways that they medicalize nonwhite facial features as aesthetically undesirable, demonstrating an underlying biopolitical desire to surgically produce a more racially homogenous nation. I was surprised at how easily a concept like the "negroid nose" could be translated into other Latin American contexts where lighter-skinned elites have a similar investment in denying indigeneity and blackness a valued place in the nation, except as folkloric representations of the past. As Julia Rodriguez points out, it is in the realms of science and medicine that racial stereotypes about Latin Americans of African or Amerindian descent are "legitimated, codified and even created," accompanied by "equally pernicious assumptions about women's capacities and the role of sexuality and reproduction in determining human worth." Rodriguez urges us to examine how these ideas are always in motion, circulating between and across national boundaries and intervening on gendered and racialized bodies in particular ways.[3]

As a regional and global center of knowledge production with regard to plastic surgery, Brazil also exports ideas about beauty, race, and nationhood that other Latin American medical experts find logical and useful. For instance, two Cuban doctors cite Brazilian literature on the "negroid nose" in an article regarding the surgical treatment of "negroid and mestizo noses" on this Caribbean island. They use a similar discourse, in which racial mixture is to blame for aesthetically unpleasing facial features, and in which plastic surgeons are able to "harmonize" patients' features through rhinoplasty.[4] They also cite, however, literature on the "mestizo nose" by Fernando Ortiz Monasterio, considered today the "father" of plastic surgery in Mexico. This suggests that Latin American plastic surgeons are in continuous dialogue across national boundaries, borrowing from one another and relying on similar assumptions about their nation's racial dynamics and the desirability of whiteness.

Medicalized racial discourses are not limited to the nose, either. The surgical technique known as bioplasty, a Brazilian invention I described in detail in chapter 6, has quickly spread across many Latin American countries despite its risks, apparently because of its purported claim to sculpt new features on any face. I easily found websites for Ecuadorian and Argentine doctors who, using language almost identical to that of Brazilian advertisements, reiterated the idea that bioplasty could create ideal "Western" features, such as prominent cheekbones and sharper jawlines.[5] This language is accompanied by pictures of white, European-looking men and women, as if to stress the underlying message that whiteness is achievable. Some surgeons have made a stronger effort to adapt the practice to their own context, such as a Peruvian plastic surgeon who, in a YouTube video, describes the "mestizo face" as characterized by "a flattened nose, a receding chin, elevated cheekbones and a soft jawline." He recommends a series of surgeries and treatments, including bioplasty, to correct these features, but is quick to point out that not everyone is unhappy with the "mestizo face" they have, and that it is simply a matter of preference.[6] On his website, this same surgeon advertises a complete facial restructuring he calls "profileplasty," and he offers the picture of a blonde white woman as the example of a "perfect face" that possesses all the right angles and measurements.[7]

I give these examples not only to demonstrate that Latin American plastic surgery has some deep-seated racial prejudices as a whole but also to suggest that we must look at the biopolitics of beauty as a transnational phenomenon, even as we pay attention to the specificity of how beauty is imagined and practiced within each context. Latin America not only shares a common preindependence history in which Spanish and Portuguese colonialism established a clear racial hierarchy that put lighter-skinned individuals at the top of the social pyramid, producing a lasting legacy of colorism, but the region also shares a postindependence neo-Lamarckian framework that understood hygienic and eugenic practices as the conduits for racial improvement, as Nancy Stepan has demonstrated.[8] Brazilian plastic surgeons, as I argued in chapter 1, inherited the eugenic aim to racially improve the nation through beautification, but they are perhaps not the only medical practitioners to have done so. It might be the case that eugenic thought is embedded throughout the entire region—which might help us explain the high rates of plastic surgery and the centrality of beauty all over Latin America.

Furthermore, beauty circulates not only through medical discourse but also through many global mediascapes that produce beauty as something to be cultivated and consumed. Returning to my ethnographic example of Priscila, I can only speculate about why the European men who sought out Priscila found her attractive, since I never got the chance to interview them, but seeking out racial difference was clearly a factor in why they joined an international dating site in the first place. The work of Jasmine Mitchell demonstrates that the racialized figure of the Brazilian mulatta is consumed not only nationally but transnationally as well, deployed by print media, films, and music videos to produce an eroticized imaginary of racial difference and tropical hypersexuality.[9] This, in turn, influences both sex tourism patterns and other international sexual liaisons between Brazilian individuals and foreigners, permeated by specific forms of racial affect.

Nonetheless, I do not want to reduce Priscila's ability to see herself in a new light to her interactions with men who perhaps fell for the racial stereotypes about Brazilian women abroad. In fact, she was very conscious that she challenged those stereotypes in important ways. There was something else happening in her outlook as a result of her travels—a new way of conceiving her relationship to her own body that came with a newfound maturity, a sense of independence, and a pride in her gender and her blackness. She told me that traveling abroad for the first time made her realize that she was not to blame for Brazilian men's devaluation of her, and that she would never again let it influence her. She said, with a smile and a playful toss of her hair, "*Agora eu sei que já sou glamorosa, meu bem*" (Now I am aware that I am already glamorous, my dear).

We can contrast the embodied understandings of the beauty that Priscila learned to see in herself, which account for intangible, affective qualities such as glamour, with the ways in which plastic surgeons reduce the body to visually diagnosable features that are in need correction or not. Rosemarie Garland-Thomson argues that there are ways of looking that produce repulsion in response to anything considered abnormal, and which distance the viewer from what he or she observes. I find that biopolitical discourses rely on a similar operation of isolating features considered ugly or different from the norm, with the purpose of rendering them perfectible. Garland-Thomson contrasts these dehumanizing ways of seeing the body with perceptions of beauty that have the ethical potential to move us toward recognizing human differences without stigmatizing others. Seeing "rare beauty" in another allows us to momentarily imagine how other bodies are lived and to feel a shared humanity that generates empathy. Thus, perceptions of beauty have the potential to be normalizing, reasserting a repetitive standard of familiarity, or to become ethical practices of inclusion.[10] When Priscila learned to see herself as glamorous, she also actively unlearned the normative ways of looking that had told her, throughout her life, that she was lacking or in excess of the norm. Her glamour, in fact, seemed to contain ineffable aspects of embodiment, such as charm and the way her body moved through physical space, rather than simply visible and quantifiable aspects of beauty.

Glamour is useful to think with because it reminds us of the alluring aspects of beauty but also of its artificiality—the archaic meaning of the English word *glamour* describes it as a magical charm or the ability to seduce someone by casting a spell. Today, to be glamorous means to personify a sense of style that others want to emulate—glamour is still seductive, but it is also contagious. Nigel Thrift argues that glamour "is a form of secular magic, conjured up by the commercial sphere," and he understands it as an affective field that traffics in aesthetic forms of pleasure across all of Western society.[11] Understanding glamour as a transnational affective field helps us understand the ways in which the ineffable qualities of embodied beauty travel from one location to the next, but I would argue that it is a global phenomenon, not simply a Western one.

Marcia Ochoa, for example, describes glamour as central to Venezuela, because it is a form of power that allows both marginalized and privileged women to conjure up forms of legibility and to translate it into affirmation or real income, always in relation to the imagined global audience of pageantry and fashion: "The production of glamour, beauty, and femininity functions within transnational economies of desire and consumption. Glamour allows its practitioners to draw down extralocal authority, to conjure a contingent space of being and belonging. However, glamour is not redemptive; it will not save you. . . . Glamour can function to create space out of hegemonic discourse, but just as easily, this space can be crushed by the power of the state, patriarchy, normativity, or colonialism."[12] Although both Ochoa and Thrift argue that glamour does a crucial form of cultural work in today's globalized world, Ochoa argues that glamour cannot be disentangled from the forms of inequality that give rise to its magic. As I argued in the introduction, magical thinking permeates the belief that beauty is a form of capital, and I suggest here that there might be a transnational aspect to the magic of glamour, tied to late capitalism's emphasis on image, celebrity culture, and the monetizing of affect.

I believe we should understand global beauty as emerging at the juncture of transnational biopolitical discourses and transnational affective fields. I am not arguing that beauty operates in the same way in different locations, but I do think we can find patterns in how glamour traverses national borders and how beauty producers borrow from one another to construct transnational discourses about what is beautiful. I do not want to give either biopolitics or affect primacy in the production of beauty, because both are necessary for beauty to matter—they represent two strands of the same cord. The difference between biopolitics and affect is that biopolitics seems to nearly always produce normative ways of looking, while affect engages both normative and nonnormative perceptions of beauty.

Priscila, for example, initially had an affective relationship to her own body that prompted her to seek the authority of medical experts to improve it, and it was only her new conception of herself as already glamorous that provided a temporary respite from that medical gaze and from the sexism and racism she suffered in Brazil. She still found pleasure, however, in her daily performances of beauty and did not have the privilege of renouncing her investment in beauty altogether. Rita Felski has argued that we should resist the impulse as feminists to dismiss the pleasures of beauty that do not lead to emancipation, because "it is far from clear that every aesthetic experience can be precisely calibrated in terms of its political consequences and effects."[13] There is an excess to affect that opens up our analysis of the pleasures and politics of beauty and allows us to embrace the paradox that practices of beauty are simultaneously empowering and disempowering.

BEYOND DOCILE BODIES

There has been a recent explosion of literature on beauty in anthropology, sociology, history, feminist theory, and cultural studies—a literature that takes beauty seriously as an object of inquiry and tries to engage with its unremitting prominence in our globalized world. Not only have beauty economies gone global through the proliferation of beauty pageants and the expansion of the fashion and cosmetic industries, but also it seems that the most negative aspects of beauty culture, too, have gone global, such as eating disorders and colorism, consolidating what Meeta Jha calls "the global beauty ideal."[14]

Nonetheless, a narrative that sees beauty as another aspect of Western imperialism or global homogenization misses the ways in which local histories and particular body politics shape how beauty emerges as a locus of concern, and why bodies come to be classified as having beauty or as lacking it. In fact, the biopolitical discourses that diagnose what an eating disorder is, in the first place, become part and parcel of how narratives about unhealthy beauty circulate to new locales, erasing the different forms of embodiment that engender particular relationships to food and to eating, as the anthropologist Rebecca Lester has argued.[15] Even practices associated with colorism, such as hair straightening and bleaching, cannot be identified as straightforward products of colonialism or a desire for hegemonic whiteness, in the opinion of scholars such as Shirley Anne Tate, because this does not account for the ways in which these practices allow black men and women to negotiate their place within the Black Atlantic, pursuing a form of "browning" that destabilizes both iconic white beauty and natural black beauty as standards to be followed.[16] In general, the argument that people's participation in beauty regimes is a form of internalized sexism and racism, or a form of self-hatred, becomes too simplistic when we give ethnographic attention to how actors on the ground experience beauty and embrace it for their own purposes.

This is not to say, however, that we should simply consider beauty to be a form of empowerment, or that there is nothing happening on a transnational level. Sarah Banet-Weiser and Laura Portwood-Stacer have pointed out that the postfeminist ideologies that embrace individual empowerment through consumption end up normalizing and even celebrating beautification regimes such as cosmetic surgery, and do nothing to disrupt dominant gender relations.[17] According to Simidele Dosekun, these postfeminist sensibilities have transnational implications as well, because they imagine cosmopolitan female consumers from the global South as empowered through practices of beauty and fashion, in contrast to impoverished women from the global South portrayed as still in need of liberation. In other words, female beauty becomes a way to reassert transnational neoliberal ideology when it becomes a measure of a country's development, and it produces a new way for people to participate in these national projects.[18]

Beauty can also enable the work of empire, as Mimi Thi Nguyen has demonstrated, when it gets deployed as part of a global human rights regime, accompanying the dubious gift of freedom. In Afghanistan, which is imagined as bereft of beauty and female agency, beauty schools were imported as part of the "civilizing process" that was supposedly designed to bring Afghani women up to date after the American military invasion.[19] For Nguyen, however, beauty is not only a form of biopower but also a promise and an imperative discourse, "one which determines what conditions are necessary to live, what forms of life are worth living, and what actions must follow to preserve, secure or replicate such forms." She also gives as an example the "Miss Landmine" beauty pageant in Cambodia, for women who have lost limbs in land-mine explosions—and she shows how the slogan of the project, "Everyone has the right to be beautiful," erases the complex history of transnational militarism that led to these land mines being set in the first place.[20]

I am struck by the similarities between this discourse about beauty in Cambodia and the one used by the Brazilian plastic surgeons to justify the expansion of their practice within the public health-care system. "The right to beauty" becomes in both cases a humanitarian gesture toward a better future, transforming beauty into a good in itself that is inextricably tied to any hope for well-being. It is a discourse that is highly gendered—it is nearly always women who need to be saved by beauty's redemptive power—and a discourse that clearly has transnational purchase as a biopolitical project. I would posit that the reason beauty's promise travels so well from one context to the next is because it crystallizes into specific regularities that feed on powerful forms of affect. Brian Massumi has argued that power structures emerge only by capturing affective tendencies and crystallizing them into self-perpetuating regularities. Massumi, in fact, prefers the term "power*ed*" structures in order to emphasize their ongoing emergence.[21] The biopolitics of beauty, applying this characterization, is also an emerging regularity that captures the transnational affective attunement to beauty as an essential value.

Biopolitics and affect are coconstituting elements that gave rise to beauty's value, producing, on the one hand, the discursive contrast between beauty and ugliness (usually lending legitimacy to other dichotomies) and, on the other hand, the visceral attachment to beauty as a form of hope. As scholars, we should pay attention to the specific instances when beauty emerges as a value, but also to the transnational elements that resurface with regularity. Mónica Moreno Figueroa and Rebecca Coleman, for example, have compared the ways in which white British girls and mestiza Mexican women experience beauty as being always compromised in the present and thus displaced to the past or deferred to the future, relying on attachments to beauty as a form of hope and optimism.[22] Both groups feel beauty in very similar ways despite the important differences in the biopolitical construction of beauty between the two countries.

When we consider beauty as a form of affect, it also helps complicate the notion that the body is a pliant or docile surface that biopolitical discourses can shape at will. Foucault himself argued in the first volume of *The History of Sexuality* that it was wrong to consider modern power to be an imposition from above, and preferred to characterize biopower as having a capillary capacity to suffuse throughout even the most private aspects of life, such as sexuality. Power, for Foucault, was a field of force relations that included both discourses and counterdiscourses, which in their circulation coproduced "reciprocal effects of power and knowledge."[23] Foucault does not specify, however, what propels biopower forward as it moves through society and saturates it with power-knowledge. Affect is the key to unlocking the reason why biopolitics, as a continuously emerging structure of power, crystallizes into certain regularities but not others. Affect helps us explain why biopower latches onto certain forms of bodily difference, providing them value, and why subjects have embodied, lived responses to biopolitical discourses. When we conceive of power structures as emerging through affect, it becomes clearer why they simultaneously feel empowering and disempowering, enabling and disabling: affect provides incipient capacity for both at all times. Paradoxically, a practice of beauty, such as a nose job, can feel like a form of self-affirmation for a patient, or can be tied to hopes of upward mobility, at the same time that it reaffirms medical knowledge about which types of beauty are racially proper.

I am not arguing, however, that resistance is always subsumed or co-opted by existing power structures. In fact, this is what always frustrated me about Foucault—there is little room in his conception of biopower for any kind of challenge to existing power structures, except through ethical forms of self-care. As Nigel Thrift argues, we need to seek a politics of hope that goes beyond Foucault, which considers the ways in which subjects are constituted not only by knowledge but also by unknowingness.[24]

In Massumi's conception, because power*ed* structures emerge through affect, they are by definition processes that can be momentarily short-circuited or redirected into new flows and directions:

> A power*ed* structure is not all-encompassing. It rises from a field of emergence that includes *it*. It is plugged into a broader field of activity on which it feeds. That field is astir with tendencies pointing to the potential for different modes of structuration. They may not amplify past the point of incipiency, they may be captured, or simply fail to take and subside back into the field of bare activity from which they came, but still their difference cannot not have been felt at some level, in some way. So even if there is no unsullied *state* of freedom to return to, there is always a *degree* of freedom offering the potential for other emergences. . . . What a body can do is trigger counter-amplifications and counter-crystallizations that defy capture by existing structures, streaming them into a continuing collective movement of escape. . . . The gesture of resistance is a micro-gesture of offered contagion, oriented otherwise than towards the structures into which the gestures of microfascism occurring on the same level, in the same field, have the tendency to channel.[25]

This is why I value small, seemingly insignificant ethnographic examples of Brazilian individuals who critique the dictatorship of beauty even as they are preparing to undergo plastic surgery themselves, or who critique the fact that beauty is distributed so unequally in society.

Ethnographic attention to beauty can provide examples of these incipient forms of critique in other locations, providing a more complex picture of how beauty is experienced around the globe. Even gestures that might be minuscule in comparison to a widespread societal approval of beauty contests and plastic surgeries can nonetheless create ripples and can emerge as viable alternatives first for individuals and then for society as a whole.

"THE FURY OF BEAUTY"

In 2007, I saw a spectacular one-person play in Rio de Janeiro that I interpret as a gesture toward resignifying beauty through affect—a play written and performed by an acclaimed black Brazilian poet and actress, Elisa Lucinda. The play, titled *Parem de Falar Mal da Rotina* (Stop Bad-Mouthing Routine), revels in the everyday routines of Lucinda's life—the small pleasures embedded in taking a shower, caring for one's hair, or choosing a dress before going out. The audience accompanies Lucinda as she navigates the intimate spaces in her home, and she addresses us directly, as if we were a close friend, or a lover in front of whom she is entirely at ease being nude, both physically and spiritually. She confesses that she loves listening in to other people's conversations, trying to piece together a story from the snippets that she catches as she takes the bus or the subway. She briefly embodies some of the absurd characters she has encountered, making us laugh. Above all, however, we witness snippets from her own routine: nothing extraordinary happens at all, and yet we feel an intimate connection with her because she is so at ease with us.

As the title of her play suggests, Lucinda's message is one of love for the ordinariness of the everyday, showcasing how simple actions such as putting on makeup or perfume contain pleasurable moments of self-affirmation. Small acts of vanity, she tells us, might seem like a drab routine, but in truth they are never exactly the same as the day before, and they always have the potential to be experienced anew, transforming the performance that is our life. Lucinda exudes a love for herself that is contagious; and as she gives us insight into the multiplicity of her day-to-day sensations, she brings to life the importance of what Kathleen Stewart calls "ordinary affects"—the seemingly banal, unremarkable patterns that nonetheless shape us as subjects, producing intensities that move between us and give us the capacity to affect and be affected.[26]

It is in this in-between, ordinary place that beauty resides and where beauty acquires value. Elisa Lucinda's play felt remarkable to me because it epitomized the ways in which beauty can be experienced as both empowering and disempowering, particularly as it circulates between and through subjects. At one point during the play, Lucinda expresses her love for her natural hair and pointedly asks her audience, "Why are you calling it *cabelo ruim* [bad hair]? This hair has never robbed anyone or hurt anyone. Has yours?" As much as Lucinda expresses love for her own body and its natural beauty, she has to engage the preconceptions in wider Brazilian culture that her natural, Afro-textured hair is not a sign of beauty but rather a sign of an unkempt appearance. She also challenges a deeper, affective association between blackness and criminality in Brazil, making the audience laugh about their own racial anxieties.

However, by the time she addresses this, she has already altered her natural hair innumerous times, using elastic hair bands to transform herself into different characters. Her hair has become a living part of Lucinda's performance, its versatility a strength that the audience cannot help but admire. Lucinda remarks on how this versatility is deadened by the compulsory norm of hair-straightening, and how women begin to lose their individuality as they seek the perfect straight hair, becoming zombielike in the long lines leading to the beauty salons. There might still be some pleasure in these normative forms of self-care, but these are routines that by definition cannot vary, cannot be experienced anew every day, and so are experienced as dictatorial. Lucinda thus demonstrates that beauty, ordinary as it is, is a way of being in the world that is paradoxically enabling and disabling at the same time, an affective quality that cannot be reduced to either structure or agency.

By defiantly asking, "Why are you calling my hair bad?" Lucinda is inserting herself within a larger, ongoing debate in Brazilian society about beauty's value and its relation to racism. The stakes of beauty are very high in Brazil, and the counterdiscourses that challenge normative definitions of beauty are still minoritarian but are growing larger by the day. Throughout this book, I have argued that beauty is a form of biopower that seeks to manage, organize, and rank the Brazilian population in a particular manner; but I was struck by the capacity of my interviewees to repopulate beauty with their own embodied experiences of social exclusion. Beauty, for them, was a lived event, something they actively felt and did in their daily lives, rather than something that was imposed on them from above. It seemed inadequate to portray beauty as an ideology that duped people into becoming willing participants, or as a rigid social structure in relation to which people acquiesce or resist. Beauty is much more than that—it is an affective quality that is felt viscerally, below the level of awareness, and something that no one has the luxury to ignore.

When Lucinda challenges us to rethink what is beautiful, she is not asking us to lift an ideological veil and pretend we are above the trappings of beauty, but is instead asking us to reevaluate the intimate and ordinary ways in which we engage with beauty, shaping who we are in relation to others. One of Elisa Lucinda's poems, "A Fúria da Beleza" (The fury of beauty), describes beauty as "a slap to the face, a gulp, a fall that paralyzes us, organizes us, disperses us, connects us and completes us."[27] Beauty is indeed unpredictable as a form of becoming, and it is also impossible to ignore—it feels like an arresting, physical impact to our body. Beauty, however, also has the power to move us, to bring us outside ourselves, and to undo us. We need to do better at explaining the hold beauty has on us, and we need new ways to theorize beauty's complex politics.

Notes

INTRODUCTION

1. Ahmed 2004: 10–11.
2. Examples of scholarship that I believe strike a good balance between agency and structure include the work of Virginia Blum (2003), Kathy Davis (2003), Victoria Pitts-Taylor (2007), Lauren Gulbas (2013), and Marcia Ochoa (2014).
3. Novaes 2006.
4. Goldenberg 2010; Edmonds 2010.
5. Edmonds 2010: 117.
6. Nguyen 2011.
7. Latour 1987.
8. Haraway 1997: 218–230.
9. Sharp 2014; Roberts 2012.
10. See, for example, the work of Adriana Petryna (2009) and Roberto Abadie (2010).
11. Martin 1998.
12. Grosz 1994: 146.
13. Butler 1993: 10.
14. Mahmood 2005.
15. Leshkowich 2014: 9.
16. Weiss 2011: 162–163.
17. Ochoa 2014: 167–169.
18. Nelson 1999: 210.
19. Mahmood 2005: 166.
20. Edmonds 2013: 79.
21. Clough 2007; Massumi 2002; Seigworth and Gregg 2010.
22. Mazzarella 2009.
23. Ahmed 2004.

24. Chen 2012.

25. Massumi 2002.

26. Clough 2005.

27. I draw from the work of Brian Massumi (2015) to model the description of power I use here.

28. Martin 2013.

29. See, for example, the work of Thomas Csordas (1993), Margaret Lock (1993), and Didier Fassin (2008).

30. Jan Slaby (2016) has described the tendency of critiques of affect theory to focus on those authors who biologize or universalize affect while they ignore the longer tradition of affect theory emerging from cultural studies, which more critically ties affect to power.

31. See the work of Emilia Sanabria (2016) for an interesting discussion on the perceived plasticity of the body in Brazil.

32. Comaroff and Comaroff 2000; Hage 2003; Piot 2010.

33. Pochmann 2012.

34. Andrea Vialli, "Mercado da beleza no Brasil deve crescer 11% em 2009," *O Estadão,* September 1, 2009.

35. "Mercado de beleza continua a crescer no Brasil, mesmo com crise," *G1,* September 7, 2015.

36. On Brazil's position as a consumer of beauty and hygiene products, see "Mercado brasileiro de cosméticos cresceu de 11% em 2014," *Brazil Beauty News,* April 17, 2015; on its position as a consumer of plastic surgery, see "Cai número de plásticas no Brasil, mas país ainda é segundo no ranking, diz estudo," *G1,* August 27, 2016.

37. Taussig 1980.

38. Taussig 1980: 136.

39. Taussig 2012.

40. On the immaterial economy's emphasis on image and surface over content, see Jameson 1990 and Harvey 1990; on that economy's emphasis on monetizing forms of affect and emotion, see Hardt and Negri 2001.

41. Ahmed 2004: 45.

42. Bourdieu 1986.

43. Bourdieu 1984: 471.

44. Grossberg 1992; Hebdige 1979; Jenkins 1992.

45. Bourdieu 1984: 193.

46. On beauty as a form of bodily capital that originates among the dominant class, see Goldenberg 2010; on beauty as a "democratizing" force, see Edmonds 2010.

47. Ahmed 2010.

48. Hordge-Freeman 2015: 103.

49. See, for example, the work of John Burdick (1998), Robin Sheriff (2001), Donna Goldstein (2003), and Kia Caldwell (2007).

50. Malysse 2002.

51. Instituto Brasileiro de Geografia e Estatística (Brazilian Institute of Geography and Statistics) website, http://seriesestatisticas.ibge.gov.br/series.aspx?vcodigo=PD336, accessed on April 14, 2017.

52. For a great analysis of the meanings of beauty practices in Salvador de Bahia, see the work of Doreen Gordon (2013).

53. On ethnographic authority, see Clifford 1983; on knowledge being always partial, see Haraway 1997; on knowledge as situated within a particular place and time, see Hall 2003.

54. For an interesting discussion of the ethics of keeping one's sexuality private in a homophobic context, see the work of Arlene Stein (2010).

55. Biehl 2005: 42–43.

1. THE EUGENESIS OF BEAUTY

1. Holston 1998.

2. Butler 1998: 28.

3. Butler 1998: 34, citing Gobineau.

4. Peixoto 1938: 42, 140, 167, italics are mine. All translations in this book are mine.

5. Stefano and das Neves 2007.

6. Romo 2010.

7. Blake 2011. I am borrowing the term *foundational fictions* from Sommer 1993.

8. Santos 2003.

9. Stepan 1991: 73.

10. Stepan 1991: 42, quoting Cruz. The 1904 Vaccine Revolt, an uprising against mandatory vaccination that almost derailed Oswaldo Cruz's sanitation campaign in Rio de Janeiro, is a small reminder of the uphill battle that Brazilian doctors experienced in their efforts to impose their authority. The medical establishment had to confront both the conservative political detractors who disagreed with the modernization policies the country was undertaking, and the popular resistance to the authoritarian intrusions of the sanitary police (see Needell 1987).

11. Penna 1918: 144, citing Chagas.

12. Rodriguez Balanta 2012.

13. Neiva and Penna 1916: plate 26.

14. Stepan 2001.

15. For more on the political dimensions of this public health campaign, see the work of José Amador (2015).

16. Pereira 1922.

17. Penna 1918: 145.

18. Penna 1918: 7.

19. Penna 1918: 107.

20. Penna 1918: 15.

21. Hochmann 1998.

22. Hochmann 1998.

23. Souza 2007: 37–39.

24. Stepan 1991: 53–54.

25. Kehl 1920a: 11–12.

26. The Brazilian League of Mental Hygiene, of which Renato Kehl, Afrânio Peixoto, and Carlos Chagas were active members, went as far as to recommend

that the state enforce sterilization for degenerate individuals, and to require prenuptial exams for engaged couples so that doctors could decide if a particular marriage would benefit national health. Such drastic measures were never instated, however, because the rapid expansion of the Brazilian economy required more laborers and not fewer, making negative eugenics an unpopular and impracticable option for the state (see Stepan 1991), and because prenuptial exams seemed unfeasible given the shortage of qualified doctors in rural areas of the country (see Otovo 2015).

27. Kehl 1920a: 15.

28. Kehl 1920a: 198–199.

29. Flores 2007: 188.

30. Anthropometry had already become extremely popular in the late nineteenth century among Brazilian criminologists, who followed the Lombrosian belief that criminals possessed measurable physiognomic differences. The sanitation movement began to use anthropometry as a way to prove that hygienic measures could indeed alter the very dimensions of the human body and create an improved workforce for the nation (see Schwarcz 1993).

31. Kehl 1920b: 10.

32. Kehl 1923: 79.

33. Sander Gilman has found evidence of plastic surgery having a similar neo-Lamarckian character within the American context, but only during the beginning of the twentieth century (Gilman 1999).

34. Kehl 1923: 421.

35. Kehl 1923: 411.

36. Kehl 1923: 167.

37. Kehl 1923: 175 and 178.

38. Paiva 2002.

39. Paiva 2002: 83, citing Irajá.

40. Irajá 1931: 19.

41. Irajá 1931: 32–33.

42. Irajá 1931: 69.

43. Irajá 1931: 86–87.

44. Some of these photographs, in fact, come from museum collections, while others are credited to an army major assigned to a command in the Amazonia state of Rondônia.

45. Linnaeus regarded Africans, Europeans, Amerindians, and Asians as belonging to four different human subspecies and as having both very different physical characteristics and different levels of intelligence. Europeans, according to him, were vastly superior to Africans (see Marks 1995: 50).

46. Irajá 1931: plate 2.

47. Irajá 1931: 47.

48. Irajá 1938: 50.

49. Irajá 1938: 159.

50. Irajá 1969.

51. De Araújo 1994; Romo 2007.

52. Freyre [1933] 2003: 375.

53. Pallares-Burke 2005.

54. Freyre [1933] 2003: 367.
55. Freyre [1933] 2003: 111.
56. Freyre [1933] 2003: 228–231.
57. Freyre [1933] 2003: 370. See also Agiar 2006.
58. Freyre [1933] 2003: 389.
59. Freyre [1933] 2003: 389.
60. Freyre [1933] 2003: 396–397.
61. Freyre [1933] 2003: 157.
62. Freyre [1933] 2003: 336–337.
63. Freyre [1933] 2003: 334.
64. Freyre [1933] 2003: 161.
65. Freyre [1933] 2003: 367.
66. Freyre [1933] 2003: 322.
67. Young 2006: 112.
68. Agiar 2006: 171.
69. Freyre 1974: 84.
70. Freyre 1966: 19.
71. Freyre 1984.
72. On Freyre's historical methodology, see Skidmore 2002; on his sanitization of slavery, see Schwarcz 1986; on his evacuation of economic relations, see Schwarcz 2006.
73. See Vianna 2000 and Lehman 2008.
74. See Dávila 2003: 213; and Weinstein 2015: 290–291.
75. Skidmore 2002.
76. Kehl 1917: 6.
77. Rebello Neto 1933.
78. Martire 2005.

2. PLASTIC GOVERNMENTALITY

1. "Senado homenageia os cirurgiões plásticos," *Agência Senado*, November 12, 2008.
2. Latour 1987.
3. Russell-Wood 1968. At the time, both this form of medical care and voting rights were limited to the white elite, which represented less than 2 percent of the total Brazilian population (Holston 2008: 102).
4. Williams 1994.
5. Menicucci 2007.
6. Lima, Fonseca, and Hochman 2005.
7. The INPS also entered into agreements with some large businesses with many employees, whereby the INPS would directly subsidize these businesses so they would provide health care to their employees, usually by subcontracting a medical provider (Menicucci 2007).
8. Menicucci 2007.
9. Escorel, Nascimento, and Edler 2005.
10. Menicucci 2007: 82.
11. Escorel, Nascimento, and Edler 2005.

12. Arretche 2005.

13. Correia 2000.

14. Noronha, Pereira, and Viacava 2005.

15. Brazilian Federation of Hospitals website, accessed on April 14, 2017, http://fbh.com.br/sobre-a-fbh/quem-somos/.

16. Fortes 2009.

17. Ong 2006.

18. Claudia Collucci, "Para frear gastos em saúde, Temer estuda rever SUS," *Folha de Sao Paulo,* August 31, 2016.

19. Fries 2008; Ilcan 2009; Lemke 2001; Nadesan 2008; Rose 2007.

20. Echeverria 1999: 80.

21. Crisóstomo, Radwanski, and Pitanguy 2004.

22. Pitanguy 1983: 63.

23. Pitanguy 1998: 75.

24. Holston 2008: 104.

25. Pitanguy, quoted in Wolfenson 2002: 62.

26. "A maior e mais espantosa tragédia ocorrida em circo," *O Globo,* December 18, 1961.

27. Maurício Joppert da Silva, "De quem é a culpa?" *O Globo,* December 28, 1961.

28. "Pele congelada para as vítimas do circo," *O Globo,* January 2, 1962.

29. Pitanguy 1983: 9–10.

30. The term *Asiatic* refers here to the indigenous population of Brazil, imagined as racially closer to Asians. The myth of origin about Brazil describes its population as the mixture of "three original races": African, Indian, and white European.

31. Foucault 1994: 83.

32. Paula Beatriz Neiva, "Marcas da violência: Agressões físicas fazem o número de cirurgias plásticas reparadoras empatar com o total de operações estéticas," *Veja,* June 12, 2002.

33. Scott 1998.

34. Travassos, personal communication, January 28, 2008.

35. Nelson 2015: 4, 23.

36. CFM *Processo-Consulta* 2003: number 641.

37. Foucault 2003: 244.

38. Nelson 2009: 238.

39. DaMatta 1986: 95–105.

40. Barbosa 1992.

41. Holston 2008.

42. Biehl 2007.

3. THE CIRCULATION OF BEAUTY

1. Wolf 1992; Balsamo 1992; Bordo 1993.

2. Davis 1995.

3. Blum 2003; Davis 2003; Pitts-Taylor 2007.

4. Ahmed 2004.

5. Grosz 1994; Clough 2000; Puar 2007.

6. Serematakis 1994: 6.

7. Allison 2013.

8. Goldenberg 2010: 220–221.

9. Edmonds 2010: 202.

10. Bourdieu 1984.

11. For more on the widespread use of muscle-building steroids in Brazil, see Sabino 2004.

12. Cohen 2004.

13. Klimpel and Whitson 2016; McCallum 2005; McCallum and dos Reis 2009; Edmonds 2010; Sanabria 2016. I, too, gave the modern too much explanatory power when I first wrote about this subject (see Jarrin 2006); but as a discourse, notions of modernity rarely came up in my interviews with patients. Plastic surgeons, however, were heavily invested in portraying their discipline as modern.

14. Chow 2010: 228.

15. See Butler (2004) for a critique of the gender-identity-disorder diagnosis in the American context, particularly as a requirement for treatment of transgender individuals.

16. Kulick 1998; Benedetti 2005.

17. A few private practices in Brazil offer surgeries to *travestis,* but most find access to surgery by traveling abroad (Vartabedian 2016).

18. Jarrin 2016.

19. Vartabedian 2016: 92–93.

20. Kulick and Machado-Borges 2005.

21. Caldwell 2007.

22. *Vix,* "O Valor da Aparência," accessed on April 18, 2017, www.vix .com/pt/bdm/dinheiro/o-valor-da-aparencia-1.

23. For a discussion of the color classification system as fluid, see Sansone 2003; on the system as ambiguous, see Telles 2006; and on the system as multiple, see Fry 1996.

24. See Burdick 1998; Caldwell 2007; Goldstein 2003; Gomes 2006; Sheriff 2001; Twine 1997.

25. Saldanha 2006; Puar 2007.

4. HOPE, AFFECT, MOBILITY

1. This narrative of upward mobility is reminiscent of the "black Cinderellas," who, Donna Goldstein (2003) argues, seek economic mobility by seducing older, white men—a more pragmatic approach than modeling, yet one crosscut by the same tendency to racialize and sexualize black women's bodies in particular ways.

2. "Da Cidade de Deus à Cidade-Luz," *Revista Tudo de Bom (Jornal O Dia),* October 2007.

3. "Conto de fadas carioca," *Jornal Extra,* October 20, 2007.

4. Ahmed 2010.

5. Gregg 2003.

6. Hardt and Negri 2004: 108–115.

7. Fortunati 2007.

8. Barrett 1988.

9. Weeks 2007.

10. Hochschild 1983.

11. Wissinger 2007.

12. Entwistle and Wissinger 2006.

13. Holston 2008.

14. Hage 2003.

15. Comaroff and Comaroff 2000.

16. Thrift 2010.

17. Hordge-Freeman 2015.

18. Mitchell 2013.

19. "Taís Araújo continua sendo a Helena mais rejeitada de todos os tempos," *Noveleiros,* March 7, 2014.

20. Araújo 2008.

21. Mankekar 1993; Abu-Lughod 2005.

22. Allison 2009.

23. Mankekar 2015.

24. Flávio Ricco, "Novela da Globo bate recorde de custo por capítulo," *Uol,* September 14, 2013. Currently three other Brazilian networks—Record, SBT, and Bandeirantes—also produce soap operas and compete with Globo for their share of the television audience.

25. Valentim 2007.

26. Hamburger 2005.

27. "Beleza na Favela," segment aired on *Hoje em Dia,* November 19, 2007.

28. "Beleza na Favela," segment aired on *Hoje em Dia,* November 19, 2007.

29. Ahmed-Ghosh 2003; Banet-Weiser 1999, 2004; Ochoa 2014.

30. "Beleza na Favela," segment aired on *Hoje em Dia,* December 10, 2008.

31. "Beleza na Favela," segment aired on *Hoje em Dia,* December 9, 2007.

32. Ochoa 2014: 32–40.

33. Jonas Pasck, "Beleza, que beleza? Na favela," *Caros Amigos,* November 25, 2008.

34. Instituto Brasileiro de Geografia e Estatística (Brazilian Institute of Geography and Statistics) website, accessed on April 14, 2017, http://seriesestatisticas .ibge.gov.br/series.aspx?vcodigo=PD336.

35. King-O'Riain 2006: 4.

36. When the model Ana Carolina Reston died of anorexia in 2006, she was portrayed in the Brazilian media as a tragic heroine who sacrificed everything to provide for her low-income family. Despite her death leading to increased awareness about anorexia, it also enshrined her sacrifice for upward mobility.

37. "Novas modelos deixam as famílias em busca do sonho das passarelas," *Profissão Repórter,* aired on June 16, 2015.

38. Dilson Stein New Models website, accessed on September 1, 2016, http:// dilsonstein.com.br/modelos_descobertos.php.

39. Daniel Targeta, "O que que as gaúchas têm? Booker fala sobre o 'borogodó' das gurias no mundo da moda," *Menina Fantástica* website, December 16, 2009, http://g1.globo.com/fantastico/quadros/menina-fantastica-2009/platb /tag/modelos/.

40. Ahmed 2010.

41. Berlant 2006: 21.

42. Sheriff 2001.

43. Goldstein 2003.

44. Edelman 2004.

45. Stewart 2007.

46. Holston 1991.

47. "Concurso da 'Garota da Laje' pára o centro do Rio," *Jornal Hoje,* aired on November 14, 2008.

48. "Candidatas da Garota da Laje param o Saara," *RJTV,* aired on November 14, 2008.

49. "A Garota da Laje," *Revista Trip,* October 24, 2003.

50. Alícia Uchôa, "Concurso Garota da Laje dá carro usado de 2001 de prêmio," *O Globo,* November 12, 2008.

51. "Concurso da 'Garota da Laje' pára o centro do Rio," November 14, 2008, *Jornal Hoje,* aired on November 14, 2008.

52. Segment of *Hoje em Dia,* aired on December 8, 2008.

53. "Concursos—Parte 1," *Profissão Repórter,* aired on July 20, 2009.

54. Kipnis 2005.

55. Edelman 2004.

56. Muñoz 2009: 7.

57. "Doze detentas participam da final do 'Miss Penitenciária' no DF," *G1,* February 28, 2008.

58. "Presa por tráfico é a beldade dos presídios," *Folha de São Paulo,* November 25, 2004.

59. "'Deusa do Ébano' do Ilê Aiyê está em filme com Mariana Ximenes," *G1,* February 13, 2010.

60. Prefeitura de Osasco website, accessed on August 6, 2015, www.osasco. sp.gov.br/belezanegra/.

61. Duggan and Muñoz 2009.

5. THE RACIOLOGY OF BEAUTY

1. Blum 2003.

2. Davis 2003: 100.

3. Gilroy 2000.

4. Wald 2006: 331–332.

5. Haraway 1997.

6. Sheriff 2001; Caldwell 2007.

7. Burdick 1998; Goldstein 2003.

8. Hordge-Freeman 2015.

9. De Santana Pinho 2009: 44.

10. Sovik 2004: 371–372.

11. Sheriff 2001: 177.

12. Chen 2012.

13. I borrow the metaphor about the viscosity of race from Saldanha (2006) and Puar (2007). See chapter 3 for an extended discussion of their work.

14. DaMatta 1986; Sansone 2003; Telles 2006; Bailey 2009; Burdick 2013.

15. Pitanguy 1993: 83.

16. Pitanguy 1993: 80. In the sanctioned English translation of the aforementioned text by Pitanguy, the word *eugenia* is replaced by the word *well-being,* perhaps illustrating that the translator was wary of how a foreign audience might regard the term.

17. "Ivo Pitanguy: O especialista em mulheres," *O Globo,* December 18, 2010.

18. "Ivo Pitanguy: O especialista em mulheres," *O Globo,* December 18, 2010.

19. BG Cirurgia Plástica website, "Rinoplastia Nariz Negróide," accessed on July 5, 2015, www.portaldacirurgiaplastica.com.br/rinoplastia-nariz-negroide/.

20. Freyre (1933) 2003: 160.

21. The category *nordestino* is a quasi-ethnic category associated with poor rural workers in northeastern Brazil, and in the Brazilian Southeast the term has acquired a negative stereotype used against dark-skinned rural migrants coming into urban areas (see Caldeira 2000).

22. Pravaz 2012.

23. Pravaz 2008.

24. The Globeleza is always black, but should also never be too black, as was made evident by a recent case where the initial winner of the contest, Nayara Justino, lost her contract with Globo owing to an onslaught of online posts that critiqued her darker hue compared to those of previous winners ("'Negra demais' para o posto, ex-Globeleza se diz 'usada' pela Globo," *Veja,* June 2, 2016).

25. Sheriff 1999.

26. Pravaz 2012.

27. Viviane Nogueira, "A fórmula das pernas perfeitas," *O Globo,* November 10, 2012.

28. "Miss Bumbum: Candidatas protestam contra prótese com formato da bunda brasileira," *Correio,* September 18, 2014.

29. "Bumbum à brasileira," *Plástica e Beleza,* December 9, 2011.

30. Manthei 2007. See also Kia Caldwell's (2007) discussion of mulattas.

31. Caldeira 2000: 70–72.

32. McClintock 1995; Chen 2012.

33. For a more extended discussion of the use of the term *crioulo* as an epithet, see Sheriff 2001.

34. Isabel Clemente, José Fucs, Solange Azevedo, and Suzane Frutuoso, "Como a violência afeta a mente e a vida de todos nós," *Época,* January 8, 2007.

35. Advertisement for the International Conference on Aesthetics, *Veja Rio,* July 26, 2006.

36. Bourdieu 1984.

37. See Karam 2008. Karam argues that this discrimination lessened recently, when Syrian-Lebanese identity was integrated into neoliberal conceptions of ideal entrepreneurship.

38. Roberts 2012.

39. Sheriff 2001.

40. Otoclinica website, "Nariz de pele grossa," accessed on July 15, 2015, www.otoclinica.com/rinoplastia/narizpelegrossa.html.

41. BG Cirurgia Plástica website, "Nariz Negróide," accessed on July 15, 2015, www.bgcirurgiaplastica.com.br/site/detalheArtigo.asp?id=67&titulo=Nariz+Negroide.

42. Hochman, de Castilho, and Ferreira 2002: 258.

43. The emphasis on anthropometry in Brazil dates back to eugenic discourses from the early twentieth century, as I explain in chapter 1.

44. Roque 1999: 91.

45. "Beleza: A perfeição é possível; Mas é desejável?" *Veja*, October 29, 2008.

46. "Beleza de boneca," *Mente Cérebro*, April 2007.

47. Caldeira 2000: 23–32.

48. Chen 2012.

49. Beatriz 2014; Araújo 2015.

50. Porfírio 2014.

6. COSMETIC CITIZENS

1. Massumi 2014.

2. Mol 2008.

3. Latour 2007; Ingold 2011.

4. "Plástica nas mãos de médicos sem especialização," *A Gazeta*, August 4, 2012.

5. "Cirurgia plástica no SUS ajuda a reconstituir a cidadania da mulher vítima da violência, diz subsecretária de Políticas para as Mulheres," *Secretaria Estadual de Direitos Humanos, Minas Gerais,* January 6, 2016.

6. Sanabria 2016: 138.

7. Rose 2007.

8. Taussig et al. 2003.

9. Rose 2007: 69–70.

10. Brandzel 2016: 5.

11. Luiz Otávio Rodrigues Ferreira, "Cirurgia plástica nos tribunais: Estética vs reparadora," *Plastikos Especial* 1 (2007): 9.

12. João Roberto Salazar, "O erro medico na perspectiva do Poder Judiciário," *Plastiko's Especial* 1 (2007): 12.

13. Dênis Calans Loma, "Prova e pericia civil e criminal na cirurgia plástica," *Plastiko's Especial* 1 (2007): 26.

14. Holston 2008. Holston also claims that Brazil's "differentiated citizenship" is being challenged by a new form of "insurgent citizenship" that produces new forms of civic participation and challenges the monopoly the wealthy have over land, but he admits that entrenched forms of inegalitarian citizenship are difficult to overturn.

15. Farmer 2004.

16. Ingold 2011: 87.

17. Mol 2002: 171.
18. Goldstein 2003.
19. Petryna 2009.
20. Petryna 2002.
21. Cohen 1999.
22. Cohen 2004: 169.
23. Abadie 2010: 72.
24. Massumi 2014: 43–45 (emphasis in the original).
25. I am borrowing the term *bioavailable* from Lawrence Cohen's (2004) description of experimental subjects.
26. Mol 2002: 179.
27. Latour 1987.
28. "Lipoaspiração é o procedimento cirúrgico que mais mata no Brasil," *iBahia,* September 13, 2016.
29. Sharp 2014.
30. Carina Rabelo and Claudia Jordão, "Exageros pela vaidade," *Istoé,* January 16, 2008.
31. "Alerta público sobre procedimento de preenchimentos estéticos," CFM press release, March 17, 2006.
32. Lipodystrophy is a condition caused by antiretroviral HIV medications and is characterized by the loss of subcutaneous fat. Since 2005, the Brazilian universal health-care system has covered the cost of bioplasty applications to treat lipodystrophy in HIV patients ("SUS amplia acesso a cirurgias reparadoras para pacientes com HIV," *Agencia Saúde,* January 23, 2009).
33. Latour 1987.
34. Martin 1998.
35. Caldeira 2000.
36. On nodules under the skin caused by PMMA, see de Jesus et al. 2015; on PMMA's migration to different tissues, see Rosa and Macedo 2001; on its migration to the liver and kidneys specifically, see Rosa et al. 2008; on blindness caused by PMMA, see Silva and Curi 2004; and on necrosis of facial tissue caused by PMMA, see de Castro et al. 2007.
37. Ingold 2012: 438.
38. Biehl 2005.
39. Fausto Carneiro, "Falta de médicos é o principal problema do SUS, mostra IPEA," *G1,* September 2, 2011.
40. "Hospitais públicos e privados sofrem com falta de pediatras," *G1,* May 2, 2016.
41. "Cortes de gastos na Saúde são 'Morte do SUS,' diz ex-Ministro," *Uol Notícias,* June 3, 2016.
42. "Prefeitura corta em até 30% o número de cirurgias eletivas em Belo Horizonte," *G1,* July 14, 2016.

CONCLUSION

1. Appadurai 1990.
2. Mitchell 2015; Williams 2013.

3. Rodriguez 2011: 428–429.

4. Canto Vidal and Canto Vigil 2010.

5. For the Ecuadorian example, see Dr. Jose Ruiz website, "Bioplastia en cara," July 21, 2015, www.joseruizecheverria.com/bioplastia/; and for the Argentine example, see MSK Center website, "Bioplastia facial," accessed on April 17, 2017, www.mskcenter.com/index.php/articulos/item/138-bioplastia-facial.

6. David Ruiz, "Rostro Mestizo," March 31, 2009, www.youtube.com /watch?v=WVqMa3wZygo.

7. David Ruiz Vela website, "Perfiloplastia," accessed on April 17, 2017, www.davidruizvela.pe/perfiloplastia/.

8. Stepan 1991.

9. Mitchell 2013.

10. Garland-Thomson 2009: 185–196.

11. Thrift 2010: 297.

12. Ochoa 2014: 89.

13. Felski 2006: 281.

14. On the proliferation of beauty pageants, see Cohen et al. 2005; on the expansion of the fashion industry, see Miller and Woodward 2011; on the expansion of the cosmetic industry, see Jones 2010; on eating disorders, see Nasser et al. 2003; on colorism, see Anekwe 2014; and on the global beauty ideal, see Jha 2015.

15. Lester 2007.

16. Tate 2012.

17. Banet-Weiser and Portwood-Stacer 2006.

18. Dosekun 2015.

19. Nguyen 2011.

20. Nguyen 2016, par. 3 and par. 8.

21. Massumi 2015.

22. Coleman and Figueroa 2010.

23. Foucault 1990: 102.

24. Thrift 2007.

25. Massumi 2015: 104–106.

26. Stewart 2007.

27. Lucinda 2006.

Bibliography

Abadie, Roberto. 2010. *The Professional Guinea Pig: Big Pharma and the Risky World of Human Subjects*. Durham, NC: Duke University Press.

Abu-Lughod, Lila. 2005. *Dramas of Nationhood: The Politics of Television in Egypt*. Chicago: University of Chicago Press.

Agiar, Michel. 2006. "Nação brasileira e mistura dos genes: As mestiçagens de Gilberto Freyre." In *Gilberto Freyre e os estudos latinoamericanos*, edited by Joshua Lund and Malcolm McNee. Pittsburgh, PA: Instituto Internacional de Literatura Latinoamericana.

Ahmed, Sara. 2004. *The Cultural Politics of Emotion*. London: Routledge.

———. 2010. *The Promise of Happiness*. Durham, NC: Duke University Press.

Ahmed-Ghosh, Huma. 2003. "Writing the Nation on the Beauty Queen's Body: Implications for a 'Hindu' Nation." *Meridians: feminism, race, transnationalism* 4 (1): 205–227.

Allison, Anne. 2009. "The Cool Brand, Affective Activism and Japanese Youth." *Theory, Culture and Society* 26 (2–3): 89–111.

———. 2013. *Precarious Japan*. Durham, NC: Duke University Press.

Amador, José. 2015. *Medicine and Nation Building in the Americas, 1980–1940*. Nashville, TN: Vanderbilt University Press.

Anekwe, Obiora N. 2014. "Global Colorism: An Ethical Issue and Challenge in Bioethics." *Voices in Bioethics: An Online Journal* (Columbia University), September 8.

Appadurai, Arjun. 1990. "Disjuncture and Difference in the Global Cultural Economy." *Theory, Culture and Society* 7 (2): 295–310.

Araújo, Clarice Fortunato. 2015. "Por que as mulheres negras são minoria no mercado matrimonial." *Geledés* (blog), May 21 post. www.geledes.org.br /por-que-as-mulheres-negras-sao-minoria-no-mercado-matrimonial/.

Araújo, Joel Zito. 2008. "O negro na dramaturgia brasileira, um caso exemplar da decadência do mito da democracia racial brasileira." *Estudos Feministas* 16 (3): 979–985.

Arretche, Marta. 2005. "A política da política de saúde no Brasil." In *Saúde e democracia: História e perspectivas do SUS*, edited by Nísia Trindade Lima, Silvia Gerschman, Flavio Coelho Edler, and Julio Manual Suárez. Rio de Janeiro: Editora Fiocruz.

Bailey, Stanley. 2009. *Legacies of Race: Identities, Attitudes and Politics in Brazil*. Stanford, CA: Stanford University Press.

Balsamo, Anne. 1992. "On the Cutting Edge: Cosmetic Surgery and the Technological Production of the Gendered Body." *Camera Obscura* 28:207–237.

Banet-Weiser, Sarah. 1999. *The Most Beautiful Girl in the World: Beauty Pageants and National Identity*. Berkeley: University of California Press.

———. 2004. "Miss America, National Identity, and the Identity Politics of Whiteness." In *"There She Is, Miss America": The Politics of Sex, Beauty and Race in America's Most Famous Pageant*, edited by Elwood Watson and Darcy Martin. New York: Palgrave Macmillan.

Banet-Weiser, Sarah, and Laura Portwood-Stacer. 2006. "'I Just Want to Be Me Again!': Beauty Pageants, Reality Television and Post-feminism." *Feminist Theory* 7 (2): 255–272.

Barbosa, Livia. 1992. *O jeitinho brasileiro: A arte de ser mais igual do que os outros*. Rio de Janeiro: Campus.

Barrett, Michele. 1988. *Women's Oppression Today: The Marxist-Feminist Encounter*. 2nd ed. London: Verso.

Beatriz, Amanda. 2014. "O padrão de beleza negra ideal." *Blogueiras Negras* (blog), April 10 post. http://blogueirasnegras.org/2014/04/10/o-padrao-de-beleza-negra-ideal/.

Benedetti, Marcos Roberto. 2005. *Toda feita: O corpo e o gênero das travestis*. Rio de Janeiro: Garamond.

Berlant, Lauren. 2006. "Cruel Optimism." *differences: A Journal of Feminist Cultural Studies* 17 (3): 20–36.

Biehl, João. 2005. *Vita: Life in a Zone of Social Abandonment*. Berkeley: University of California Press.

———. 2007. *Will to Live: AIDS Therapies and the Politics of Survival*. Princeton, NJ: Princeton University Press.

Blake, Stanley E. 2011. *The Vigorous Core of Our Nationality: Race and Regional Identity in Northeastern Brazil*. Pittsburgh, PA: University of Pittsburgh Press.

Blum, Virginia. 2003. *Flesh Wounds: The Culture of Cosmetic Surgery*. Berkeley: University of California Press.

Bordo, Susan. 1993. *Unbearable Weight: Feminism, Western Culture, and the Body*. Berkeley: University of California Press.

Bourdieu, Pierre. 1984. *Distinction: A Social Critique of the Judgment of Taste*. Cambridge, MA: Harvard University Press.

———. 1986. "The Forms of Capital." In *Handbook of Theory and Research for the Sociology of Education*, edited by John G. Richardson. New York: Greenwood.

Brandzel, Amy. 2016. *Against Citizenship: The Violence of the Normative.* Chicago: University of Illinois Press.

Burdick, John. 1998. *Blessed Anastácia: Women, Race and Popular Christianity in Brazil.* New York: Routledge.

———. 2013. *The Color of Sound: Race, Religion and Music in Brazil.* New York: New York University Press.

Butler, Judith. 1993. *Bodies That Matter: On the Discursive Limits of "Sex."* New York: Routledge.

———. 2004. *Undoing Gender.* New York: Routledge.

Butler, Kim D. 1998. *Freedoms Given, Freedoms Won: Afro-Brazilians in Post-abolition São Paulo and Salvador.* New Brunswick, NJ: Rutgers University Press.

Caldeira, Teresa Pires do Rio. 2000. *City of Walls: Crime, Segregation and Citizenship in São Paulo.* Berkeley: University of California Press.

Caldwell, Kia Lilly. 2007. *Negras in Brazil: Re-envisioning Black Women, Citizenship and the Politics of Identity.* New Brunswick, NJ: Rutgers University Press.

Canto Vidal, Bernaldo, and Tania Canto Vigil. 2010. "Rinoplastia en la nariz mestiza y negroide: Una preocupación de todos." *Medisur* 8 (1): 26–31.

CFM *Processo-Consulta.* 2000–2008. Archives at the Conselho Regional de Medicina do Estado de Rio de Janeiro (CREMERJ). Rio de Janeiro, Brazil.

Chen, Mel Y. 2012. *Animacies: Biopolitics, Racial Mattering and Queer Affect.* Durham, NC: Duke University Press.

Chow, Rey. 2010. "The Elusive Material: What the Dog Doesn't Understand." In *New Materialisms: Ontology, Agency and Politics*, edited by Diana Coole and Samantha Frost. Durham, NC: Duke University Press.

Clifford, James. 1983. "On Ethnographic Authority." *Representations* 1 (2): 118–146.

Clough, Patricia Ticineto. 2000. *Autoaffection.* Minneapolis: Minnesota University Press.

———. 2005. "The Affective Turn: Political Economy and the Biomediated Body." Seminar presented at the University of Leicester.

———. 2007. Introduction to *Theorizing the Social*, edited by Patricia Ticineto Clough and Jean Halley. Durham, NC: Duke University Press.

Cohen, Colleen Ballerino, Richard Wilk, and Beverly Stoeltje, eds. 1996. *Beauty Queens on the Global Stage: Gender, Contests, and Power.* New York: Routledge.

Cohen, Lawrence. 1999. "Where It Hurts: Indian Material for an Ethics of Organ Transplantation." *Daedalus* 128 (4): 135–165.

———. 2004. "Operability: Surgery at the Margin of the State." In *Anthropology in the Margins of the State*, edited by Veena Das and Deborah Poole. New Delhi: Oxford University Press.

Coleman, Rebecca, and Mónica Moreno Figueroa. 2010. "Past and Future Perfect? Beauty, Affect and Hope." *Journal for Cultural Research* 14 (4): 357–373.

Comaroff, Jean, and John L. Comaroff. 2000. "Millenial Capitalism: First Thoughts on a Second Coming." *Public Culture* 12 (2): 291–343.

Correia, Maria Valéria Costa. 2000. *Que controle social? Os conselhos de sáude como instrumento*. Rio de Janeiro: Editora Fiocruz.

Crisóstomo, Márcio, with Henrique Radwanski and Ivo Pitanguy. 2004. "Importância da 38ª Enfermaria da Santa Casa da Misericórdia do Rio de Janeiro para a Cirurgia Plástica Brasileira." *Revista do Médico Residente* 6 (4): 44–47.

Csordas, Thomas. 1993. "Somatic Modes of Attention." *Cultural Anthropology* 8 (2): 135–156.

DaMatta, Roberto. 1986. *O que faz o brasil, Brasil?* Rio de Janeiro: Rocco.

Dávila, Jerry. 2003. *Diploma of Whiteness: Race and Social Policy in Brazil, 1917–1945*. Durham, NC: Duke University Press.

Davis, Kathy. 1995. *Reshaping the Female Body: The Dilemma of Cosmetic Surgery*. New York: Routledge.

———. 2003. *Dubious Equalities and Embodied Differences: Cultural Studies on Cosmetic Surgery*. Lanham, MD: Rowman and Littlefield.

de Araújo, Ricardo Benzaquen. 1994. *Guerra e paz: Casa Grande e Senzala e a obra de Gilberto Freyre nos anos 30*. Rio de Janeiro: Editora 34.

de Castro, Anderson Castelo Branco, Marcus Vinicius Martins Collares, Ciro Paz Portinho, Paulo Cesar Dias, and Rinaldo de Angeli Pinto. 2007. "Necrose facial extensa após infiltração com polimetilmetacrilato." *Revista Brasileira de Otorrinolaringologia* 73 (6): 850.

de Jesus, Luciano Henrique, Laura de Campos Hildebrand, Manoela Domingues Martins, Francine Miranda da Rosa, Chris Krebs Danilevicz, and Manoel Sant'Ana Filho. 2015. "Location of Injected Polymethylmethacrylate Microspheres Influences the Onset of Late Adverse Effects: An Experimental and Histopathologic Study." *Clinical, Cosmetic and Investigational Dermatology* 8:431–436

de Santana Pinho, Patricia. 2009. "White but Not Quite: Tones and Overtones of Whiteness in Brazil." *Small Axe* 13 (2): 39–56.

Dosekun, Simidele. 2015. "For Western Girls Only? Post-feminism as Transnational Culture." *Feminist Media Studies* 15 (6): 960–975.

Duggan, Lisa, and José Muñoz. 2009. "Hope and Hopelessness: A Dialogue." *Women and Performance: A Journal of Feminist Theory* 19 (2): 275–283.

Echeverria, Regina. 1999. *Ivo Pitanguy: O Mestre da Beleza*. Coleção Gente do Século. São Paulo: Editora Três.

Edelman, Lee. 2004. *No Future: Queer Theory and the Death Drive*. Durham, NC: Duke University Press.

Edmonds, Alexander. 2010. *Pretty Modern: Beauty, Sex and Plastic Surgery in Brazil*. Durham, NC: Duke University Press.

———. 2013. "The Biological Subject of Aesthetic Medicine." *Feminist Theory* 14 (1): 65–82.

Entwistle, Joanne, and Elizabeth Wissinger. 2006. "Keeping Up Appearances: Aesthetic Labour in the Fashion Modeling Industries of London and New York." *Sociological Review* 5 (4): 774–794.

Escorel, Sarah, Dilene Raimundo do Nascimento, and Flavio Coelho Edler. 2005. "As origens da reforma sanitária e do SUS." In *Saúde e democracia: História e perspectivas do SUS*. Rio de Janeiro: Editora Fiocruz.

Farmer, Paul. 2004. *Pathologies of Power: Health, Human Rights, and the New War on the Poor.* Berkeley: University of California Press.

Fassin, Didier. 2008. "The Embodied Past: From Paranoid Style to Politics of Memory in South Africa." *Social Anthropology* 16 (3): 312–328.

Felski, Rita. 2006. "'Because It Is Beautiful': New Feminist Perspectives on Beauty." *Feminist Theory* 7 (2): 273–282.

Flores, Maria Bernardete Ramos. 2007. *Tecnologia e estética do racismo: Ciência e arte na política da beleza.* Chapecó: Argos.

Fortes, Alexandre. 2009. "In Search of a Post-Neoliberal Paradigm: The Brazilian Left and Lula's Government." *International Labor and Working-Class History* 75 (Spring): 109–125.

Fortunati, Leopoldina. 2007. "Immaterial Labor and Its Machinization." *ephemera: theory & politics in organization* 7 (1): 139–157.

Foucault, Michel. 1990. *The History of Sexuality.* Vol. 1: *An Introduction.* New York: Vintage.

———. 1994. *The Birth of the Clinic: An Archeology of Medical Perception.* New York: Random House Vintage Books.

———. 2003. *The Essential Foucault.* Edited by Paul Rabinow and Nikolas Rose. New York: New Press.

Freyre, Gilberto. [1933] 2003. *Casa grande e senzala: Formação da família brasileira sob o regime da economia patriarcal.* Recife: Global Editora.

———. 1966. *The Racial Factor in Contemporary Politics.* Vol. 1, published for the Research Unit for the Study of Multi-Racial Societies at the University of Sussex. Brighton, U.K.: MacGibbon and Kee.

———. 1974. *The Gilberto Freyre Reader.* Translated by Barbara Shelby. New York: Alfred A. Knopf.

———. 1984. "Bunda: Paixão Nacional." *Playboy,* no. 113 (December).

Fries, Christopher J. 2008. "Governing the Health of the Hybrid Self: Integrative Medicine, Neoliberalism, and the Shifting Biopolitics of Subjectivity." *Health Sociology Review* 17 (4): 353–367.

Fry, Peter. 1996. "O que a Cinderela Negra tem a dizer sobre a 'política racial' no Brasil." *Revista USP* (São Paulo), (28): 122–135.

Garland-Thomson, Rosemarie. 2009. *Staring: How We Look.* Oxford: Oxford University Press.

Gilman, Sander L. 1999. *Making the Body Beautiful: A Cultural History of Aesthetic Surgery.* Princeton, NJ: Princeton University Press.

Gilroy, Paul. 2000. *Against Race: Imagining Political Culture beyond the Color Line.* Cambridge, MA: Harvard University Press.

Goldenberg, Mirian. 2010. "The Body as Capital: Understanding Brazilian Culture." *Vibrant—Virtual Brazilian Anthropology* 7 (1): 220–238.

Goldstein, Donna. 2003. *Laughter out of Place: Race, Class, Violence and Sexuality in a Rio Shantytown.* Berkeley: University of California Press.

Gomes, Nilma Lino. 2006. *Sem perder a raiz: Corpo e cabelo como símbolos da identidade negra.* Belo Horizonte: Auténtica.

Gordon, Doreen. 2013. "A beleza abre portas: Beauty and the Racialized Body among Black Middle-Class Women in Salvador, Brazil." *Feminist Theory* 14 (2): 203–218.

Gregg, Jessica. 2003. *Virtually Virgins: Sexual Strategies and Cervical Cancer in Recife, Brazil.* Stanford: Stanford University Press.

Grossberg, Lawrence. 1992. *We Gotta Get Out of This Place: Popular Conservatism and Postmodern Culture.* New York: Routledge.

Grosz, Elizabeth. 1994. *Volatile Bodies: Towards a Corporeal Feminism.* Bloomington, IN: Indiana University Press.

Gulbas, Lauren E. 2013. "Embodying Racism: Race, Rhinoplasty and Self-Esteem in Venezuela." *Qualitative Health Research* 23 (3): 326–335.

Hage, Ghassan. 2003. *Against Paranoid Nationalism: Searching for Hope in a Shrinking Society.* London: Merlin Press.

Hall, Stuart. 2003. "Cultural Identity and Diaspora." *Theorizing Diaspora: A Reader,* edited by Jana Evans Braziel and Anita Mannur. Malden, MA: Blackwell.

Hamburger, Esther Império. 2005. *O Brasil antenado: A sociedade da novela.* Rio de Janeiro: Jorge Zahar Editora.

Haraway, Donna. 1997. *Modest_Witness@Second_Millenium.Femaleman_ Meets_ Oncomouse: Feminism and Technoscience.* New York: Routledge.

Hardt, Michael, and Antonio Negri. 2001. *Empire.* Cambridge, MA: Harvard University Press.

———. 2004. *Multitude.* New York: Penguin.

Harvey, David. 1990. *The Condition of Postmodernity: An Enquiry into the Origins of Cultural Change.* Cambridge, MA: Blackwell.

Hebdige, Dick. 1979. *Subculture: The Meanings of Style.* London: Routledge.

Hochman, Bernardo, Helton Traber de Castilho, and Lydia Masako Ferreira. 2002. "Padronização fotográfica e morfométrica na fotogrametria computarizada do nariz." *Acta Cirúrgica Brasileira* 17 (4): 258–266.

Hochman, Gilberto. 1998. "Logo ali, no final da avenida: *Os Sertões* redefinidos pelo movimento sanitarista da Primeira República." *História, Ciências, Saúde—Manguinhos* 5 (July): S217–235.

Hochschild, Arlie Russell. 1983. *The Managed Heart: Commercialization of Human Feeling.* Berkeley: University of California Press.

Holston, James. 1991. "Autoconstruction in Working-Class Brazil." *Cultural Anthropology* 6 (4): 447–465.

———. 2008. *Insurgent Citizenship: Disjunctions of Democracy and Modernity in Brazil.* Princeton, NJ: Princeton University Press.

Hordge-Freeman, Elizabeth. 2015. *The Color of Love: Racial Features, Stigma and Socialization in Black Brazilian Families.* Austin: University of Texas Press.

Ilcan, Suzan. 2009. "Privatizing Responsibility: Public Sector Reform under Neoliberal Government." *Canadian Review of Sociology* 46 (3): 207–234.

Ingold, Tim. 2011. *Being Alive: Essays on Movement, Knowledge and Description.* London: Routledge.

———. 2012. "Toward an Ecology of Materials." *Annual Review of Anthropology* 41:427–442.

Irajá, Hernani de. 1931. *Morphologia da mulher: A plástica feminina no Brasil.* Rio de Janeiro: Freitas Bastos.

———. 1938. *Sexo e beleza.* 3rd ed. Rio de Janeiro: Edição Getúlio Costa.

———. 1969. *Sexo e virgindade: Reconstituição da virgindade física*. Rio de Janeiro: Editora Pongetti.

Jameson, Fredric. 1992. *Postmodernism, or, the Cultural Logic of Late Capitalism*. Durham, NC: Duke University Press.

Jarrin, Alvaro. 2006. "The Right to Beauty: Cosmetic Citizenship and Medical Modernity in Brazil." *Exchange: Journal of the Anthropology Department at the University of Chicago.* http://ucexchange.uchicago.edu/articles/theRightToBeauty.html.

———. 2016. "Untranslatable Subjects: Travesti Access to Public Health Care in Brazil." *TSQ: Transgender Studies Quarterly* 3 (3–4): 357–375.

Jenkins, Henry. 1992. *Textual Poachers: Television Fans and Participatory Culture*. New York: Routledge.

Jha, Meeta. 2015. *The Global Beauty Industry: Colorism, Racism, and the National Body*. London: Routledge.

Jones, Geoffrey. 2010. *Beauty Imagined: A History of the Global Beauty Industry*. Oxford: Oxford University Press on Demand.

Karam, John Tofik. 2008. *Another Arabesque: Syrian-Lebanese Ethnicity in Neoliberal Brazil*. Philadelphia, PA: Temple University Press.

Kehl, Renato. 1917. "A eugenia: Sciencia do aperfeiçoamento moral e physico dos seres humanos." Paper presented at the Associação Cristã de Moços in São Paulo, April 13.

———. 1920a. *Eugenia e Medicina Social (problemas da vida)*. Rio de Janeiro: Livraria Francisco Alves.

———. 1920b. *Povo são e povo doente: Algumas consideracões a dados anthropométricos*. Rio de Janeiro: Brazil-Medico.

———. 1923. *A cura da fealdade: Eugenia e medicina social*. São Paulo: Monteiro Lobato and Editores.

———. 1936. *A fada hygia: Primeiro livro de higiene (Adoptado officialmente pela Diretoria Geral de Instrução Pública de varios Estados do Paiz)*. Rio de Janeiro: Livraria Francisco Alves.

King-O'Riain, Rebecca Chiyoko. 2006. *Pure Beauty: Judging Race in Japanese American Beauty Pageants*. Minneapolis: University of Minnesota Press.

Kipnis, Laura. 2005. "(Male) Desire and (Female) Disgust: Reading Hustler." *Popular Culture: A Reader*, edited by Raiford Gins and Omayra Zaragoza Cruz. London: Sage Publications.

Klimpel, Jill, and Risa Whitson. 2016. "Birthing Modernity: Spatial Discourses of Cesarean Birth in São Paulo, Brazil." *Gender, Place and Culture* 23 (8): 1207–1220.

Kulick, Don. 1998. *Travesti: Sex, Gender and Culture among Brazilian Transgendered Prostitutes*. Chicago: University of Chicago Press.

Kulick, Don, and Thais Machado-Borges. 2005. "Leaky." In *Fat: The Anthropology of an Obsession*. New York: Jeremy P. Tarcher/Penguin.

Lacerda, João Batista. 1911. *Sur les métis au Brésil*. Paris: Imprimerie Devouge.

Latour, Bruno. 1987. *Science in Action: How to Follow Scientists and Engineers through Society*. Cambridge, MA: Harvard University Press

———. 2007. *Reassembling the Social: An Introduction to Actor-Network Theory*. Oxford: Oxford University Press.

Lehman, David. 2008. "Gilberto Freyre: A reavaliação prossegue." *Horizontes Antropológicos* 14 (29): 369–385.

Lemke, Thomas. 2001. "'The Birth of Bio-Politics': Michel Foucault's Lecture at the College de France on Neo-liberal Governmentality." *Economy and Society* 30 (2): 190–207.

Leshkowich, Ann Marie. 2014. *Essential Trade: Vietnamese Women in a Changing Marketplace.* Honolulu: University of Hawaii Press.

Lester, Rebecca J. 2007. "Critical Therapeutics: Cultural Politics and Clinical Reality in Two Eating Disorder Treatment Centers." *Medical Anthropology Quarterly* 21 (4): 369–387.

Lima, Nísia Trindade, Cristina Fonseca, and Gilberto Hochman. 2005. "A saúde na construção do Estado Nacional no Brasil: Reforma sanitária em perspectiva histórica." In *Saúde e democracia: História e perspectivas do SUS*, edited by Nísia Trindade Lima, Silvia Gerschman, Flavio Coelho Edler and Julio Manual Suárez. Rio de Janeiro: Editora Fiocruz.

Lock, Margaret. 1993. "Cultivating the Body: Anthropology and Epistemologies of Bodily Practice and Knowledge." *Annual Review of Anthropology* 22:133–155.

Lucinda, Elisa. 2006. *A fúria da beleza.* Rio de Janeiro: Editora Record.

Mahmood, Saba. 2005. *Politics of Piety: The Islamic Revival and the Feminist Subject.* Princeton, NJ: Princeton University Press.

Malysse, Stéphane. 2002. "Em busca dos (H)alteres-ego: Olhares franceses ons bastidores da corpolatria carioca." In *Nu and Vestido: Dez antropólogos revelam a cultura do corpo carioca*, edited by Mirian Goldenberg. Rio de Janeiro: Editora Record.

Mankekar, Purnima. 1993. "National Texts and Gendered Lives: An Ethnography of Television Viewers in a North Indian City." *American Ethnologist* 20 (3): 543–563.

———. 2015. *Unsettling India: Affect, Temporality, Transnationality.* Durham, NC: Duke University Press.

Manthei, Jennifer. 2007. "The Brazilian *Mulata*: A Wood for All Works." *Negotiating Identities in Modern Latin America*, edited by Hendrik Kaay. Calgary: University of Calgary Press.

Marks, Jonathan. 1995. *Human Biodiversity: Genes, Race and History.* New York: Aldine Transaction.

Martin, Emily. 1998. "Anthropology and the Cultural Study of Science." *Science, Technology and Human Values* 23 (1): 24–44.

———. 2013. "The Potentiality of Ethnography and the Limits of Affect Theory." *Current Anthropology* 54 (7): S149–S258

Martire, Lybio, Jr. 2005. "História da cirurgia plástica brasileira." In *Cirurgia Plástica*, edited by Sergio Carreirão, Vera Cardim, Dov Goldenberg. São Paulo: Editora Atheneu.

Marx, Karl. 1992. *Capital.* Vol. 1: *A Critique of Political Economy.* New York: Penguin Classics.

Massumi, Brian. 2002. *Parables for the Virtual: Movement, Affect, Sensation.* Durham, NC: Duke University Press.

———. 2014. *The Power at the End of the Economy*. Durham, NC: Duke University Press.

———. 2015. *Politics of Affect*. Cambridge, U.K.: Polity Press.

Mazzarella, William. 2009. "Affect: What Is It Good For?" *Enchantments of Modernity: Empire, Nation, Globalization*, edited by Saurabh Dube. London: Routledge.

McCallum, Cecilia. 2005. "Explaining Cesarean Section in Salvador da Bahia, Brazil." *Sociology of Health and Illness* 27 (2): 215–242.

McCallum, Cecilia, and Ana Paula dos Reis. 2009. "Passagem solitária: Parto hospitalar como ritual em Salvador da Bahia, Brasil." In *Demografia em Debate*. Vol. 2, edited by Paulo Miranda-Ribeiro and Andréa Branco Simão. Belo Horizonte: Associação Brasileira de Estudos Populacionais.

McClintock, Anne. 1995. *Imperial Leather: Race, Gender and Sexuality in the Colonial Conquest*. New York: Routledge.

Menicucci, Telma Maria Gonçalves. 2007. *Público e privado na política de assistência à saúde no Brasil: Atores, processos e trajetória*. Rio de Janeiro: Editora Fiocruz.

Miller, Daniel, and Sophie Woodward, eds. 2011. *Global Denim*. Oxford: Berg.

Mitchell, Gregory. 2015. *Tourist Attractions: Performing Race and Masculinity in Brazil's Sexual Economy*. Chicago: University of Chicago Press.

Mitchell, Jasmine. 2013. "Popular Culture Imaginings of the Mulatta: Constructing Race, Gender, and Nation in the United States and Brazil." PhD diss., University of Minnesota.

Mol, Annemarie. 2002. *The Body Multiple: Ontology in Medical Practice*. Durham, NC: Duke University Press.

———. 2008. *The Logic of Care: Health and the Problem of Patient Choice*. London: Routledge.

Muñoz, José. 2009. *Cruising Utopia: The Then and There of Queer Futurity*. New York: NYU Press.

Nadesan, Majia Holmer. 2008. *Governmentality, Biopower and Everyday Life*. New York: Routledge.

Nasser, Mervat, Melanie Katzman, and Richard Gordon, eds. 2003. *Eating Disorders and Cultures in Transition*. London: Routledge.

Needell, Jeffrey D. 1987. "The *Revolta Contra Vacina* of 1904: The Revolt against 'Modernization' In *Belle-Époque* Rio de Janeiro." *Hispanic American Historical Review* 67 (2): 233–269.

Neiva, Arthur, and Belisário Penna. 1916. "Viagem científica pelo norte da Bahia, sudoeste do Pernambuco, sul do Piauhí e de norte a sul do Goiaz." *Memórias do Instituto Oswaldo Cruz* (Rio de Janeiro) 8 (3): 74–224.

Nelson, Diane M. 1999. *A Finger in the Wound: Body Politics in Quincentennial Guatemala*. Berkeley: University of California Press.

———. 2009. *Reckoning: The Ends of War in Guatemala*. Durham, NC: Duke University Press.

———. 2015. *Who Counts?: The Mathematics of Death and Life after Genocide*. Durham, NC: Duke University Press.

Nguyen, Mimi Thi. 2011. "The Biopower of Beauty: Humanitarian Imperial-isms and Global Feminisms in an Age of Terror." *Signs* 36 (2): 359–383.

———. 2016. "The Right to Be Beautiful." *The Account: A Journal of Poetry, Prose and Thought.* www.theaccountmagazine.com/article/the-right-to-be-beautiful.

Noronha, José de Carvalho, with Telma Ruth Pereira and Francisco Viacava. 2005. "As condições de saúde dos brasileiros: Duas décadas de mudanças (1980–2000)." In *Saúde e democracia: História e perspectivas do SUS,* edited by Nísia Trindade Lima, Silvia Gerschman, Flavio Coelho Edler, and Julio Manual Suárez. Rio de Janeiro: Editora Fiocruz.

Novaes, Joana de Vilhena. 2006. *O intolerável peso da feiura: Sobre as mulheres e seus corpos.* Rio de Janeiro: Editora PUC/Garamond.

Ochoa, Marcia. 2014. *Queen for a Day: Transformistas, Beauty Queens and the Performance of Femininity in Venezuela.* Durham, NC: Duke University Press.

Ong, Aihwa. 2006. *Neoliberalism as Exception: Mutations in Citizenship and Sovereignty.* Durham, NC: Duke University Press.

Otovo, Okezi T. 2015. "Marrying 'Well': Debating Consanguinity, Matrimonial Law, and Brazilian Legal Medicine, 1890–1930." *Law and History Review* 33 (3): 703–743.

Paiva, Sabrina Pereira. 2002. "A difusão da sexologia no Brasil na primeira metade do século XX: Um estudo sobre a obra de Hernani de Irajá." Master's thesis, Instituto de Medicina Social, UERJ.

Pallares-Burke, Maria Lúcia Garcia. 2005. *Gilberto Freyre: Um vitoriano nos trópicos.* São Paulo: Editora Unesp.

Peixoto, Afrânio. 1938. *Clima e saúde: Introdução biogeográfica à civilização brasileira.* São Paulo: Companhia Editora Nacional.

Penna, Belisário. 1918. *Saneamento do Brasil: Sanear o Brasil é povoal-o, é enriquecel-o, é moralisal-o.* Rio de Janeiro: Typografia Revista dos Tribunaes.

Pereira, Miguel. 1922. "O Brasil ainda é um immenso hospital." *Revista da Medicina* 3 (22): 3–9.

Petryna, Adriana. 2002. *Life Exposed: Biological Citizens after Chernobyl.* Princeton, NJ: Princeton University Press.

———. 2009. *When Experiments Travel: Clinical Trials and the Global Search for Human Subjects.* Princeton, NJ: Princeton University Press.

Piot, Charles. 2010. *Nostalgia for the Future: West Africa after the Cold War.* Chicago: University of Chicago Press.

Pitanguy, Ivo. 1983. *Direito à Beleza: Memórias do grande mestre da cirurgia plástica.* Rio de Janeiro: Editora Record.

———. 1993. "Criatividade e cirurgia plástica." *Revista Brasileira de Cirurgia* 83 (2): 79–86. Rio de Janeiro: Cidade-Editora Científica Ltda.

———. 1998. "Especial: Ivo Helcio Jardim de Campos Pitanguy." *Médicos,* special issue.

Pitts-Taylor, Victoria. 2007. *Surgery Junkies: Wellness and Pathology in Cosmetic Culture.* New Brunswick, NJ: Rutgers University Press.

Pochmann, Márcio. 2012. *Nova classe média?: O trabalho na base da pirâmide social brasileira.* São Paulo: Boitempo Editorial.

Porfírio, Gabi. 2014. "Racismo disfarçado de ciência." *Blogueiras Negras* (blog), March 6 post. http://blogueirasnegras.org/2014/03/06/racismo-disfarcado-de-ciencia/.

Pravaz, Natasha. 2008. "Where Is the Carnivalesque in Rio's Carnival? Samba, Mulatas and Modernity." *Visual Anthropology* 21 (2): 95–111.

———. 2012. "Performing *Mulata*-ness: The Politics of Cultural Authenticity and Sexuality among Carioca Samba Dancers." *Latin American Perspectives* 39 (2): 113–133.

Puar, Jasbir K. 2007. *Terrorist Assemblages: Homonationalism in Queer Times.* Durham, NC: Duke University Press.

Rebello Neto, José. 1933. "Da cirurgia estética em face da responsabilidade legal." *Revista Brasileira de Otorrinolaringologia* 1 (1): 23–45.

Roberts, Elizabeth F. S. 2012. *God's Laboratory: Assisted Reproduction in the Andes.* Berkeley: University of California Press.

Rodriguez, Julia. 2011. "A Complex Fabric: Intersecting Histories of Race, Gender, and Science in Latin America." *Hispanic American Historical Review* 91 (3): 409–429.

Rodriguez Balanta, Beatriz Eugenia. 2012. "Especimenes antropometricos y curiosidades pintorescas: La orquestacion fotografica del cuerpo negro (Brasil circa 1865)." *Revista Ciencias de la Salud* 10 (2): 223–242.

Romo, Anadelia A. 2007. "Rethinking Race and Culture in Brazil's First Afro-Brazilian Congress of 1934." *Journal of Latin American Studies* 39:31–54.

———. 2010. *Brazil's Living Museum: Race, Reform and Tradition in Bahia.* Chapel Hill: University of North Carolina Press.

Roque, Carlos. 1999. *Magos da beleza: Conceitos e visões de nove cirurgiões plásticos brasileiros.* Brasil: Edição do Autor.

Rosa, Simone Corrêa, and Jefferson Lessa Soares de Macedo. 2001. "Reações adversas a substâncias de preenchimento subcutâneo." *Revista Brasileira de Cirurgia Plástica* 20 (4): 248–252.

Rosa, Simone Corrêa, Albino Verçosa de Magalhães, and Jefferson Lessa Soares de Macedo. 2008. "An Experimental Study of Tissue Reaction to Polymethyl Methacrylate (PMMA) Microspheres (Artecoll) and Dimethylsiloxane (DMS) in the Mouse." *American Journal of Dermatopathology* 30 (3): 222–227.

Rose, Nikolas. 2007. *The Politics of Life Itself: Biomedicine, Power, and Subjectivity in the Twenty-First Century.* Princeton, NJ: Princeton University Press.

Russell-Wood, A. J. R. 1968. *Fidalgos and Philanthropists: The Santa Casa da Misericórdia of Bahia, 1550–1755.* Berkeley: University of California Press.

Sabino, Cesar. 2004. "O peso da forma: Cotidiano e uso de drogas entre fisiculturistas." PhD diss., Universidade Federal do Rio de Janeiro, 2004.

Saldanha, Arun. 2006. "Reontologizing Race: The Machinic Geography of Phenotype." *Environment and Planning D: Society and Space* 24 (1): 9–24.

Sanabria, Emilia. 2016. *Plastic Bodies: Sex Hormones and Menstrual Suppression in Brazil.* Durham, NC: Duke University Press.

Sansone, Livio. 2003. *Blackness without Ethnicity: Constructing Race in Brazil.* New York: Palgrave Macmillan.

Santos, Ricardo Augusto dos. 2003. "Lobato, os Jecas e a questão racial no pensamento social brasileiro." *Achegas.net* 1 (7), www.achegas.net/numero /sete/ricardo_santos.htm.

Scheper-Hughes, Nancy. 1992. *Death without Weeping: The Violence of Everyday Life in Brazil.* Berkeley: University of California Press.

Schwarcz, Lilia Moritz. 1993. *O espetáculo das raças: Cientistas, instituições e questão racial no Brasil, 1870–1930.* São Paulo: Companhia das Letras.

———. 2006. "Gilberto Freyre: Adaptação, mestiçagem, trópicos e privacidade em *Novo Mundo nos trópicos.*" In *Gilberto Freyre e os estudos latinoamericanos,* edited by Joshua Lund and Malcolm McNee. Pittsburgh, PA: Instituto Internacional de Literatura Latinoamericana.

Schwarcz, Stuart B. 1986. *Sugar Plantations in the Formation of Brazilian Society: Bahia, 1550–1835.* Cambridge, MA: Cambridge University Press.

Scott, James C. 1998. *Seeing Like a State: How Certain Schemes to Improve the Human Condition Have Failed.* New Haven, CT: Yale University Press.

Seigworth, Gregory J., and Melissa Gregg. 2010. "An Inventory of Shimmers." In *The Affect Theory Reader,* edited by Melissa Gregg and Gregory J. Seigworth. Durham, NC: Duke University Press.

Seremetakis, C. Nadia. 1994. *The Senses Still: Perception and Memory as Material Culture in Modernity.* Chicago: Chicago University Press.

Sharp, Lesley A. 2014. *The Transplant Imaginary: Mechanical Hearts, Animal Parts and Moral Thinking in Highly Experimental Science.* Berkeley: University of California Press.

Sheriff, Robin E. 1999. "The Theft of Carnaval: National Spectacle and Racial Politics in Rio de Janeiro." *Cultural Anthropology* 14 (1): 3–28.

———. 2001. *Dreaming Equality: Color, Race and Racism in Urban Brazil.* New Brunswick, NJ: Rutgers University Press.

Silva, Marcus Tulius T., and André Land Curi. 2004. "Blindness and Total Ophthalmoplegia after Aesthetic Polymethylmethacrylate Injection: Case Report." *Arquivos de neuro-psiquiatria* 62 (3B): 873–874.

Skidmore, Thomas. 1993. *Black into White: Race and Nationality in Brazilian Thought.* Durham, NC: Duke University Press.

———. 2002. "Raízes de Gilberto Freyre." *Journal of Latin American Studies* 34 (1): 1–20.

Slaby, Jan. 2016. "Relational Affect." Working Paper SFB 1171, Affective Societies 02/16, Freie Universitat Berlin, Berlin. www.diss.fu-berlin.de/docs /servlets/MCRFileNodeServlet/FUDOCS_derivate_000000006442 /SFB1171_WP_02–16.pdf.

Sommer, Doris. 1993. *Foundational Fictions: The National Romances of Latin America.* Berkeley: University of California Press.

Souza, Vanderlei Sebastião de. 2007. "Em nome da raça: A propaganda eugênica e as ideias de Renato Kehl nos anos 1910 e 1920." *Revista de História Regional* 11 (20): 29–70.

Sovik, Liv. 2004. "Aqui ninguém é branco: Hegemonia branca e *media* no Brasil." In *Branquidade: Identidade branca e multiculturalismo,* edited by Vron Ware. Rio de Janeiro: Garamond.

Stefano, Waldir, and Marcia das Neves. 2007. "Mestiçagem e eugenia: Um estudo comparativo entre as concepções de Raimundo Nina Rodrigues e Otavio Domingues." *Filosofia e História da Biologia* 2:445–456.

Stein, Arlene. 2010. "Sex, Truths and Audiotape: Anonymity and the Ethics of Exposure in Public Ethnography." *Journal of Contemporary Ethnography* 39 (5): 554–568.

Stepan, Nancy Leys. 1991. *"The Hour of Eugenics": Race, Gender, and Nation in Latin America*. Ithaca, NY: Cornell University Press.

———. 2001. *Picturing Tropical Nature*. Ithaca, NY: Cornell University Press.

Stewart, Kathleen. 2007. *Ordinary Affects*. Durham, NC: Duke University Press.

Tate, Shirley Anne. 2012. *Black Beauty: Aesthetics, Stylization, Politics*. London: Ashgate.

Taussig, Karen-Sue, Deborah Heath, and Rayna Rapp. 2003. "Flexible Eugenics: Technologies of the Self in the Age of Genetics." In *Genetic Nature/Culture*, edited by A.H. Goodman, D. Heath and M.S. Lindee. Berkeley: University of California Press.

Taussig, Michael. 1980. *The Devil and Commodity Fetishism in South America*. Chapel Hill: University of North Carolina Press.

———. 2012. *Beauty and the Beast*. Chicago: University of Chicago Press.

Telles, Edward. 2006. *Race in Another America: The Significance of Skin Color in Brazil*. Princeton, NJ: Princeton University Press.

Thrift, Nigel. 2007. "Overcome by Space: Reworking Foucault." In *Space, Knowledge and Power: Foucault and Geography*, edited by Jeremy W. Crampton and Stuart Elden. London: Ashgate.

———. 2010. "Understanding the Material Practices of Glamour." In *The Affect Theory Reader*, edited by Melissa Gregg and Gregory J. Seigworth. Durham, NC: Duke University Press.

Twine, France Winddance. 1997. *Racism in a Racial Democracy: The Maintenance of White Supremacy in Brazil*. New Brunswick, NJ: Rutgers University Press.

Valentim, Aldo Luiz. 2007. *Internacionalização da Rede Globo: Estudo de caso da exportação de telenovelas*. São Paulo: Centro Universitário das Faculdades Metropolitanas Unidas.

Vartabedian, Julieta. 2016. "Beauty That Matters: Brazilian *Travesti* Sex Workers Feeling Beautiful." *Sociologus* 66 (1): 73–96.

Vianna, Hermano. 2000. "Equilíbrio de antagonismos." *Folha de São Paulo*, March 12.

Wald, Priscilla. 2006. "Blood and Stories: How Genomics Is Rewriting Race, Medicine and human history." *Patterns of Prejudice* 40: 4, 303–333.

Weeks, Kathi. 2007. "Life within and against Work: Affective Labor, Feminist Critique, and Post-Fordist Politics." *ephemera: theory & politics in organization* 7 (1): 233–249.

Weinstein, Barbara. 2015. *The Color of Modernity: São Paulo and the Making of Race and Nation in Brazil*. Durham, NC: Duke University Press.

Weiss, Margot. 2011. *Techniques of Pleasure: BDSM and the Circuits of Sexuality*. Durham, NC: Duke University Press.

Williams, Erica Lorraine. 2013. *Sex Tourism in Bahia: Ambiguous Entanglements*. Chicago: University of Illinois Press.

Williams, Steven C. 1994. "Prelude for Disaster: The Politics and Structures of Urban Hygiene in Rio de Janeiro, 1808–1860." PhD diss. University of California, Los Angeles.

Wissinger, Elizabeth. 2007. "Modelling a Way of Life: Immaterial and Affective Labour in the Fashion Modelling Industry." *ephemera: theory & politics in organization* 7 (1): 250–269.

Wolf, Naomi. 1992. *The Beauty Myth: How Images of Beauty Are Used against Women*. New York: Doubleday.

Wolfenson, Moisés. 2002. *Transformações: Arte and Cirurgia Plástica*. Rio de Janeiro: Editora Revan.

Young, Robert J. C. 2006. "O Atlântico lusotropical: Gilberto Freyre e a transformação do hibridismo." *Gilberto Freyre e os estudos latino-americanos*, edited by Joshua Lund and Malcom McNee. Pittsburgh: Instituto Internacional de Literatura Latinoamericana.

Index

Fig. refers to figures

CPSIA information can be obtained
at www.ICGtesting.com
Printed in the USA
LVHW091443310720
662059LV00002B/459